Allergy: the unmet need

A blueprint for better patient care

A report of the Royal College of Physicians Working Party
on the provision of allergy services in the UK

Royal College of Physicians

June 2003

Royal College of Physicians of London
11 St Andrews Place, London NW1 4LE

Registered charity No. 210508

Copyright © 2003 Royal College of Physicians of London

ISBN 1 86016 183 9

Cover design: Merriton Sharp

Typeset by Dan-Set Graphics, Telford, Shropshire

Printed in Great Britain by The Lavenham Press Ltd, Sudbury, Suffolk

Contents

PART TWO

Allergy: a brief guide to causes, diagnosis and management

Members of the Working Party

Stephen T Holgate MD DSc FRCP FRCPE FIBiol FRCPath FMedSci *(Chair)*, MRC Clinical Professor of Immunopharmacology, School of Medicine, University of Southampton

Pamela W Ewan MA MB FRCP FRCPath *(Deputy Chair)*, Consultant in Allergy and Honorary Lecturer, Addenbrooke's Hospital, University of Cambridge Clinical School

Anthony P Bewley MB ChB FRCP, Consultant in Dermatology, Whipps Cross Hospital, London

Carol M Black CBE ND PRCP, President, Royal College of Physicians

Jonathan Brostoff DM DSc(Med) FRCP FRCPath FIBiol, Senior Research Fellow, Professor Emeritus of Allergy and Enviromental Health, King's College London

Christine Carter BSc SRD, Specialist Paediatric Dietitian, Great Ormond Street Hospital for Children, London

John W Coleman BSc PhD, Reader, Department of Pharmacology and Therapeutics, University of Liverpool

Paul Cullinan MB FRCP, Senior Lecturer, Department of Occupational and Environmental Medicine, Imperial College National Heart and Lung Institute, London

Adnan Custovic PhD DM MD, Professorial Clinical Research Fellow, North West Lung Centre, Wythenshawe Hospital, Manchester

Stephen R Durham MA MD FRCP, Professor of Allergy and Respiratory Medicine, Faculty of Medicine, Imperial College National Heart and Lung Institute, London

Jean Emberlin PhD, Director, National Pollen Research Unit, University College Worcester

Anthony J Frew MD FRCP, Professor of Allergy and Respiratory Medicine, School of Medicine, University of Southampton

G John Gibson MD FRCP FRCPE, Professor of Respiratory Medicine, University of Newcastle upon Tyne

Ian T Gilmore MB FRCP, Registrar, Royal College of Physicians

Julian M Hopkin MD MSc FRCP FRCPE, Professor of Medicine and Director of the Clinical School, University of Wales Swansea

Peter H Howarth DM FRCP, Consultant Allergist, Southampton General Hospital

A Barry Kay PhD DSc FRCP FRCPE FRCPath FRSE FMedSci, Professor of Allergy and Clinical Immunology, Imperial College National Heart and Lung Institute, London

M Thirumula Krishna MB PhD MRCP MRCPath, Specialist Registrar in Allergy, Southampton General Hospital

Gideon Lack BM BCH FRCPCH, Consultant in Paediatric Allergy and Immunology, St Mary's Hospital, London

Tak H Lee MA MD ScD FRCP FRCPath FMedSci, Head of Division, Department of Asthma, Allergy and Respiratory Science, Guy's, King's and St Thomas' School of Medicine, London

Roy E Pounder MD DSc(Med) FCRP, Clinical Vice President, Royal College of Physicians

Richard J Powell DM FRCP FRCPath, Reader and Consultant Physician in Allergy and Clinical Immunology, University Hospital, Queen's Medical Centre, Nottingham

David Reading Director, Anaphylaxis Campaign, Farnborough, Hants

Dermot Ryan MB MRCGP RCPI DCH, General Practitioner, Woodbrook Medical Centre, Loughborough; Clinical Research Fellow, University of Aberdeen

Samantha Walker RGN PhD, Director of Research, National Respiratory Training Centre, Warwick

John O Warner MD FRCP FRCPCH, Professor of Child Health, Southampton General Hospital

Those who were consulted

H Ross Anderson MD FRCP, Professor of Public Health Medicine, St George's Hospital Medical School, London

Peter S Friedmann MD FRCP FMedSci, Professor of Dermatology, School of Medicine, University of Southampton

Jeffrey M Graham MA PhD FFPHM, Department of Health

Ramyani Gupta MSc, Epidemiologist, Lung and Asthma Information Agency, St George's Hospital Medical School, London

Phil Hannaford MD FRCGP MFFP MFPHM DRCOG DCH, Grampian Health Board Chair of Primary Care; Director of Institute of Applied Health Sciences, University of Aberdeen; Department of General Practice and Primary Care, University of Aberdeen

Mark L Levy MBChB FRCGP, General Practitioner, Harrow; Senior Lecturer, Department of Primary Care and General Practice, Aberdeen University

MS Shuaib Nasser MD MCRP, Consultant in Allergy and Asthma, Addenbrooke's Hospital, Cambridge

David Price MA MB DRCOG MRCGP, General Practice Airways Group Professor of Primary Care Respiratory Medicine, Department of General Practice and Primary Care, University of Aberdeen

Aziz Sheikh MD MSc MRCP MRCGP, NHS R&D National Primary Care Post Doctoral Fellow, St George's Hospital Medical School, London

Colin Simpson MSc PhD, Research Fellow, Department of General Practice and Primary Care, University of Aberdeen

David Strachan MD FRCP FFPHM MRCGP, Professor of Epidemiology, St George's Hospital Medical School, London

Stephen Wasserman MD, Professor of Medicine, University of San Diego, California

Xiaohong Zheng MSc PhD, Research Assistant, Department of General Practice and Primary Care, University of Aberdeen

Foreword

Allergy is a major public health problem in developed countries. In the UK over the last twenty years, the incidence of common allergic diseases has trebled, giving this country one of the highest rates of allergy in the world. In any one year, 12 million people in the UK (one-fifth of the population) are now likely to be seeking treatment for allergy. Potentially life-threatening but previously rare allergies, such as peanut allergy which now affects one in 70 children, are increasing. But despite the epidemic proportions of the disease, the health service is failing to meet the most minimal standards of care – far less clinical governance.

This report shows clearly that there are far too few specialist allergists to meet the needs of the population, either in terms of delivering direct care in dedicated allergy centres, or in providing training for other specialists, general practitioners and practice nurses. It should be possible for milder cases of allergy to be recognised and treated in primary care so that only the more severe and complex cases need referral to a consultant. However, without the appropriate infrastructure and training this is not possible – and the health service will continue to fail to keep pace with the needs of allergy patients.

In publishing this report, the Royal College of Physicians aims to put allergy higher on the healthcare agendas of the Department of Health and planners and managers. We have made proposals for a much improved allergy service which, given the will to change and understanding of the problems faced by allergy patients, will result in more consultants, a network of accessible centres around the country, and much improved and wider training of those who care for patients. These proposals require urgent action.

June 2003

Professor Carol Black
President,
Royal College of Physicians

Preface

Allergic disease is one of the major causes of illness in developed countries and its prevalence is increasing steadily. In the UK, allergic disease affects about one in three of the population. In 13- to 14-year-old children, 32% report symptoms of asthma, 9% have eczema, and 40% have allergic rhinitis.[1] The UK ranks highest in the world for asthma symptoms, with a prevalence 20-fold higher than that of Indonesia, and is also near the top of the world ranking for allergic rhinitis and eczema.[1,2] High and increasing trends are also apparent in nut allergy,[3,4] anaphylaxis,[5,6] occupational allergy (eg latex),[7] and allergic reactions to drugs.[8]

Although genetic susceptibility is an important risk factor for allergic sensitisation and its expression as disease in different organs, the current allergy 'epidemic' is a consequence of our changing environment. Increased exposure to allergens and air pollutants, over-use of antibiotics and other drugs, reduced fruit and vegetable intake, reduced early life exposure to bacterial products, and an alteration in bacterial colonisation of the gut have all been blamed.

Allergy is an important branch of medicine and specialisation is required to provide a high-quality service for the diagnosis and treatment of allergic disease.[9] Unfortunately, in the UK such a service has not developed. Allergic disease now causes problems of increased complexity and commonly involves several organ systems,[10] so patients are often referred to a succession of different specialists, resulting only in confusion. Instead, a single referral to an allergy specialist would be both effective and cost saving. General practices and hospitals usually have little, if any, resources for establishing the presence (or absence) of sensitisation to specific allergens. In consequence, most allergic disease is treated with drugs, with little attention being paid to establishing causative agents and allergen avoidance strategies.

There is a major shortage of allergy specialists, with only six fully staffed allergy clinics in the UK, that have developed mainly around research interests. Allergy barely features in the undergraduate medical curriculum, and the lack of specialists means virtually no clinical training is available. Opportunities for postgraduate clinical training are limited. Knowledge of good allergy management in practice is therefore minimal or non-existent.

The allergy charities, along with NHS Direct, are inundated with telephone enquiries from a public desperate for help with their allergy problems. The severity of their symptoms, with attendant high morbidity, has forced the public to look outside the NHS. This has led to the proliferation of dubious allergy practice in the field of complementary and alternative medicine, where unproven techniques for diagnosis and treatment are used.[11,12] In 1992, the Royal College of Physicians (RCP) produced a report, *Allergy: conventional and alternative concepts*,[13] which drew attention to the importance of good clinical practice in allergy and the dangers of relying on practitioners of complementary and alternative medicine to deliver a competent allergy service to the public. In 1994, this was reinforced by a second report, *Good allergy practice: standards of care for providers and purchasers of allergy services within the NHS*.[14] Although both reports were well received, their impact on improving the provision of allergy services in the NHS has been limited.

The impact of allergic disease, the dearth of NHS services, and wide differences in disease management across the UK created the impetus for this third RCP report. In drawing attention to the high and ever-increasing prevalence and complexity of allergy, the disease burden this creates, and the lack of any cohesive approach to delivering an adequate clinical service within the NHS, this report highlights the unmet needs of the many patients who suffer from allergy, and the impaired quality of life that they endure.[4,15] With the influence that the public now exerts over their healthcare, the increase in multi-professional working, and the political will to provide further resources for the NHS, the time has come to make a determined effort to improve clinical services for patients with allergic disease in the UK.

June 2003

Stephen T Holgate
Pamela W Ewan

References

1   The International Study of Asthma and Allergies in Childhood (ISAAC) Steering Committee. Worldwide variation in prevalence of symptoms of asthma, allergic rhinoconjunctivitis, and atopic eczema: ISAAC. *Lancet* 1998;**351**:1225–32.

2   European Community Respiratory Health Survey. Variations in the prevalence of respiratory symptoms, self-reported asthma attacks, and use of asthma medication in the European Community Respiratory Health Survey (ECRHS). *Eur Respir J* 1996;**9**:687–95.

3   Tariq SM, Stevens M, Matthews S, Ridout S *et al.* Cohort study of peanut and tree nut sensitisation by age of 4 years. *BMJ* 1996;**313**:514–17.

4   Grundy J, Matthews S, Bateman B, Dean T, Arshad SH. Rising prevalence of allergy to peanut in children: data from 2 sequential cohorts. *J Allergy Clin Immunol* 2002;**110**:784-9.

5   Ewan PW. Anaphylaxis. *BMJ* 1998;**316**:1442–5.

6   Sheikh A, Alves B. Hospital admissions for anaphylaxis: time trend study. *BMJ* 2000;**320**:1441.

7   Garabrant DH, Schweitzer S. Epidemiology of latex sensitization and allergies in health care workers. *J Allergy Clin Immunol* 2002:**110**:582–95 (Review).

8   Demoly P, Bousquet J. Epidemiology of drug allergy. *Curr Opin Allergy Clin Immunol* 2001:**1**;305–10.

9   Pepys J. 'Clinical immunology' and the 'practise of allergy'. *Clin Allergy* 1971;**1**:1–7.

10 Bousquet J. Allergy as a global problem: 'Think globally, act globally'. *Allergy* 2000;**57**:661–2.

11 Bielory L. 'Complementary and alternative medicine' population based studies: a growing focus on allergy and asthma. *Allergy* 2002;**57**:6455–8.

12 Schäfer T, Riehle A, Wichmann H-E, Ring J. Alternative medicine in allergies: prevalence, patterns of use and costs. *Allergy* 2002;**57**:694–700.

13 Royal College of Physicians. *Allergy: conventional and alternative concepts.* Report of the Royal College of Physicians Committee on Clinical Immunology and Allergy. London: RCP, 1992.

14 Royal College of Physicians and Royal College of Pathologists. *Good allergy practice: standards of care for providers and purchasers of allergy services within the NHS.* London: RCP, 1994.

15 Van Vijk RG. Allergy: a global problem. Quality of life. *Allergy* 2002;**47**:1097–110.

Executive summary and recommendations

Background

This report discusses the implications for the NHS of the dramatic increase in allergy in recent years, including severe life-threatening and multi-system allergies. Drawing on recent research on the prevalence of allergic disease in the UK, it reveals the gulf between the need for effective advice and treatment and the lack of appropriate professional services, and proposes a strategy to address this. There is an urgent need for these proposals to be implemented, given that the incidence of allergy and related diseases is almost certain to continue to rise. The report is therefore addressed to the Department of Health, primary care trusts, hospital trusts, as well as all healthcare professionals involved in allergy care, including those in primary care.

Allergy and allergy specialists

Allergy specialists deal with a wide range of disorders, such as rhinitis, asthma, urticaria, angioedema (including hereditary angioedema), eczema, anaphylaxis, and allergy to food, drugs, latex rubber and venom. They also have the expertise to exclude allergy as a diagnosis, allowing the patient to proceed with other appropriate investigations.

The above disorders may result from generation of IgE antibody (allergic antibody), but the same disorders and symptoms, eg anaphylaxis, drug or food allergy, can occur through mechanisms that are independent of IgE. Whilst symptoms may be restricted to one organ – for example the nose in hay fever – in many allergic disorders there are systemic effects that involve several different sites in the body.

Allergy specialists undergo a long period of training to acquire the knowledge and experience needed to correctly diagnose and treat both IgE- and non-IgE-mediated allergies.

An increasing problem

Allergy is an increasing problem in the UK for three main reasons:

Increased incidence The incidence of allergy has increased dramatically in the UK in recent years and is still rising. Recent studies put the rise as approximately three-fold in the last 20 years, giving the UK one of the highest rates of allergic disease in the world. The latest estimates suggest that one-third of the total UK population – approximately 18 million people – will develop allergy at some time in their lives.

Increased severity The nature of allergic disease has also changed, so a number of severe and potentially life-threatening disorders, which were previously rare, are now common. As part of the increase in incidence, more children are now affected, particularly by previously little-known food allergies, such as peanut allergy. These are also among the most serious allergies, and accurate diagnosis, advice and treatment are vital.

Increased complexity Another development is that patients now usually have disorders affecting several systems. For example, a child with peanut allergy often also has eczema, rhinitis and asthma – so-called 'multi-system allergic disease'. Poorly controlled asthma in a patient with nut allergy is a risk factor for life-threatening or fatal reactions.

The following statistics, taken from the body of the report, illustrate these changes (some of these statistics are underestimates, since allergy can remain undiagnosed):

▶ Asthma, rhinitis and eczema have increased in incidence two- to three-fold in the last 20 years.

▶ Anaphylaxis, a severe and potentially life-threatening reaction, occurs in over one in 3,500 of the population each year as a result of exposure to substances to which the sufferer is allergic. Hospital admissions because of anaphylaxis have increased seven-fold over the last decade and doubled over four years.

▶ Food allergy is increasingly common and is the most common cause of anaphylaxis in children. Peanut allergy, the most common food allergy to cause fatal or near-fatal reactions, has trebled in incidence over four years and now affects one in 70 children in the UK. Yet only 10 years ago this was a rare disorder.

▶ Drug allergy is also increasingly common. Adverse drug reactions account for 5% of all hospital admissions in the UK. Up to 15% of inpatients have a hospital stay prolonged as a result of drug allergy. These figures do not include the majority of drug allergies, which occur in primary care and remain undiagnosed and unrecorded.

▶ Some 8% of healthcare workers now have an allergy to latex rubber, which in some cases can lead to anaphylaxis. Yet until 1979 only two cases of latex allergy had been reported.

▶ Allergic disease currently accounts for 6% of general practice consultations, 0.6% of hospital admissions, and 10% of the GP prescribing budget. The cost (in primary care, excluding hospital services) to the NHS is £900 million per annum.

Current deficits in NHS allergy services

Responsibility for the treatment of allergic disease in the NHS is shared between GPs and hospital services. However, there are three major problems:

1   Even before the recent increases in the incidence of allergic disease, there was a shortage of specialists with the expertise required to give the necessary advice and treatment, and to lead the search for ways to contain the 'epidemic':

▶ **Across the whole country, only six major centres staffed by consultant allergists offer a full-time service with expertise in all types of allergic problems. A further nine centres staffed by allergists offer a part-time service.**

▶ The remaining allergy clinics in the UK – the majority – are run part-time by consultants in other disciplines. However, they do not have the facilities to cope with the rising tide of allergies or with the problems posed by severe or multi-system allergic disorders.

▶ **There is a marked geographical inequality in service provision,** as most allergy specialists are based in London and the south-east. Services are extremely poor in the rest of the country.

▶ Overall, the provision of consultant allergists is approximately one per 2 million of the UK population, compared with rates of around one per 100,000 for mainstream specialties such as gastroenterology, cardiology, etc.

2   Allergy services in hospitals have traditionally been provided by different specialists according to the organ system affected; for example, allergic asthma is often managed by chest physicians, allergic skin disorders by dermatologists, and allergic rhinitis by ENT specialists. However, **most organ-based specialists have no training in allergy**. In addition, the development of severe, multi-system and non-organ-based disorders means that allergy now has to be considered as a health issue in its own right.

3   Currently, many allergy cases are dealt with by GPs, but because allergy has only recently become such a major problem, **the majority of GPs have no clinical training in allergy**. Furthermore, the shortage of specialists means that GPs often have no ready source of expert advice. The skill base needed to develop allergy services which are led directly from primary care is currently absent.

As a result of the problems outlined above, patients generally find great difficulty in obtaining good advice on allergy. The health service lacks the infrastructure to close the gap between needs and services. Thus, the most common reasons for calls to helplines run by allergy charities, eg the Anaphylaxis Campaign or Allergy UK, are:

▶   'My GP does not know about allergy.'

▶   'There is no allergy service near me.'

▶   'The "allergy clinic" I was referred to did not know how to help me.'

A strategy for addressing the problems

1   Allergy needs a 'whole system' approach in which allergy is treated as a condition in its own right, and not as a series of diseases depending on the organ system involved.

2   The number of allergy specialists is totally insufficient to meet the need. Proper provision of allergy specialists would mean better access, diagnosis and advice for patients, and would provide a knowledge base from which primary carers could develop their services.

3   A more effective partnership is required between allergy specialists and the primary carers, who will need to provide the bulk of the day-to-day support for people with allergy. A hub-spoke network with allergists supporting GPs and organ-based and other specialists in local hospitals should be developed.

Recommendations

The recommendations set out in this report are intended to form the basis for the development of a coordinated service over the coming decade. It is envisaged that such a service will progressively become primary care led, with expertise available from the hospital setting for more severe and complex problems. However, given the current lack of training and knowledge in primary care, initially an allergy service would need to be led by allergy specialists. It follows that there must first be an increase in numbers of allergy consultants, as detailed below. Within the hospital sector, the increase in multi-system and severe allergic disease indicates the need for consultant allergists who can provide a 'one-stop-shop' approach for patients.

General recommendations for an improved allergy service

1   The provision of allergy care in the NHS must be led by specialists trained in allergy so that appropriate standards of care can be achieved and maintained. Given the scale of what amounts to a national epidemic, the front line for allergy management must be within primary care. However, with virtually no primary care skill base to work from, clinical leadership must come initially from specialist centres. They will need to take on the dual role of diagnosis and management of the most complex cases, and of supporting the development of capacity within primary care.

2   The NHS therefore needs to move forward on two fronts. As an essential first step, more consultant posts and funded training posts in allergy are required. Specialist allergists must become the core leadership for a national training and clinical development initiative for the whole service. They must also provide the essence of a genuinely national allergy service for the NHS. The creation of these posts, and their appropriate service development context, requires a recognition of need by the Department of Health, the Workforce Numbers Advisory Board, primary care trusts, regional commissioners and trust managers.

3   The report proposes the setting up of appropriately staffed regional allergy centres evenly distributed across the whole country. Based on the service models which exist in those parts of the UK fortunate enough to have established specialist centres, they will give equality of access to appropriate allergy services for adults and children in all parts of the country. They will also provide expertise and lead the development of other local services, networking with organ-based specialists and GPs.

4   Regional commissioning for specialist allergy must also be implemented. This will require central direction.

The specific recommendations of the report are grouped below under five headings.

Specific recommendations

Regional allergy centres

5   The working party endorses the recommendations of the British Society for Allergy and Clinical Immunology (BSACI) that **each of the eight NHS Regions in England (as configured in 2001, each with a population of approximately 5–7 million), as well as Scotland, Wales and Northern Ireland, should have an absolute minimum of one regional specialist allergy centre.**

6   Staffing levels required to set up a new regional centre or develop an existing one are as follows:

   ▶ a minimum of two new/additional (whole time equivalent) consultant allergists (for adult services) offering a multidisciplinary approach. This is the minimum requirement to provide necessary cover for diagnostic procedures and specialist treatment.

   ▶ a minimum of two full-time allergy nurse specialists

   ▶ one half-time adult dietitian and one half-time paediatric dietitian with specialist training in food allergy

   ▶ two consultants in paediatric allergy, supported by paediatric nurse specialists and dietitians with expertise in paediatric allergy

   ▶ facilities for training for two specialist registrars in allergy (in some centres).

7   The regional centres should:

- ▶ provide specialist expertise for adult and paediatric allergic disease throughout their Region (tertiary care), including allergic disorders recognised for regional commissioning

- ▶ manage allergic disease in the local population which cannot be dealt with in general practice (secondary care)

- ▶ act as an educational resource for the Region

- ▶ network with and facilitate local training in allergy for organ-based specialists and paediatricians

- ▶ support training at local level for GPs and nurses in the management of common allergies in primary care.

Trainees in allergy

8   **In order to create new consultant posts, it is essential to increase the number of trainees in the specialty.** There are now only five trainees nationally.

9   The lack of trainees is creating a planning blight, because NHS trusts wishing to create new consultant posts cannot readily find suitable applicants. The Department of Health and the Workforce Numbers Advisory Board must recognise the need and provide for more funded training posts in allergy. Despite the pressing case for an increase in specialist registrar numbers, and a provisional agreement for seven additional funded posts, allergy has been allocated no new funded posts for 2003–5.

Other consultant posts in allergy

10   **In addition to regional allergy centres, further consultant allergist posts need to be created in other teaching hospitals** and district general hospitals in each Region to deal with local needs. All teaching hospitals should have an allergy service provided by a consultant allergist. One model might be for a shared appointment between trusts. This should follow the establishment of regional centres.

Training in allergy for primary care

11   Primary care must ultimately provide the front line care for allergy but considerable development is needed.

12   **The training of GPs and practice nurses in allergy needs to be improved.** A key part of this will follow from interaction with consultant allergists, and the inclusion of clinical allergy training in the undergraduate medical curriculum. There are currently a number of allergy courses for GPs and practice nurses, eg through the National Respiratory Training Centre, Southampton University, or one-day training courses run by the BSACI. However, a much more comprehensive nationwide approach is needed, covering primary care training across the NHS. The development of general practitioners with a special interest (GPSIs) in allergy, trained in and linked to regional centres, should support this.

Organ-based specialists with an interest in allergy

13   Organ-based specialists will continue to contribute to allergy care and have primary responsibility for patients with asthma and eczema, in patients with single-organ involvement. They should network with the specialist allergist who can act as a resource in identifying/ managing allergy. The increase in allergy means that greater awareness of the contribution of allergy in these organ-based specialties is important.

Summary

The NHS is currently not coping with the size and nature of the problems presented by allergy and related conditions. In order to develop a coherent model of service delivery, which would eventually be primary care based but networked to specialist allergists, major allergy centres must first be developed in all parts of the country. This requires the urgent creation of more consultant posts and training posts in allergy. These are key to:

► the improvement of patient care

► the prevention of severe and fatal allergic reactions

► the development of a coordinated allergy service

► understanding and containing the allergy 'epidemic'.

PART ONE

Allergy services: current deficits and recommendations for improvement

1. What is allergy?

1.1   Allergy is a form of exaggerated sensitivity (hypersensitivity) to a substance which is either inhaled, swallowed, injected, or comes into contact with the skin, eye or mucosa. The term 'allergy' is used for situations where hypersensitivity results from heightened (or 'altered') reactivity of the immune system in response to external or 'foreign' substances. Foreign substances that provoke allergies are called allergens. Examples include grass, weed and tree pollens, substances present in house dust (particularly the house dust mite), fungal spores, animal products, certain foods, and various chemical agents found in the home and at work.

1.2   Patients who develop common allergies such as hay fever are called 'atopic'. The common atopic diseases are listed in Box 1.1. The atopic state runs in families and is genetically transmitted. Atopic individuals produce increased amounts of the allergic antibody immunoglobulin E (IgE), a type of antibody which binds particularly strongly to mast cells. When the cell-associated IgE is 'cross-linked' by the specific allergen to which it is directed, the mast cells become activated to release inflammatory pro-allergic chemicals such as histamine and leukotrienes (see Fig. 1.1). Histamine causes the acute symptoms of allergy, ie sneezing, itching, rash, tissue swelling or fall in blood pressure, whereas leukotrienes cause airway

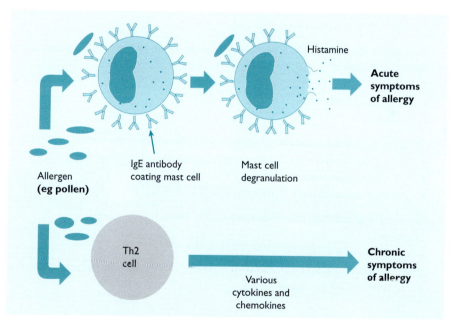

Fig 1.1   A diagrammatic representation of the basic mechanisms in the common atopic allergic diseases, ie those involving IgE, mast cells and Th2 cells. Allergen interacts with IgE bound to mast cells to cause the acute symptoms of allergy through the release of histamine and other mediators (eg leukotrienes). IgE is a Y-shaped molecule. The long arm of the Y is the part that binds avidly to the surface of the mast cell. The short arm links with the allergen in a 'lock and key' fashion. Here, pollen, the cause of hay fever, is given as an example of the allergen. When pollen binds with IgE, it triggers a series of biochemical events leading to the release of histamine and other substances which cause the symptoms of allergy. This process is sometimes called 'mast cell degranulation' because the granules, which contain the histamine, are released outside the cell. The Th2 cell is believed to play a central role in ongoing chronic symptoms by synthesising inflammatory proteins called cytokines and chemokines.

Box 1.1 Categories of allergy and its mimics

Category 1 Classical atopic disease

- Allergic rhinitis (including hay fever)
- Allergic (atopic) asthma
- Immediate (IgE-mediated) reactions to foods, eg nuts, eggs, fresh fruit
- Anaphylaxis, eg foods, insect stings, drugs
- Urticaria
- Angioedema
- Atopic eczema
- Food allergy
- Drug allergy
- Venom allergy
- Latex allergy

Some of the above may be occupational

Category 2 Non-IgE-mediated disorders managed by an allergist

Some types of:

- Rhinitis
- Urticaria, eg idiopathic and physical
- Drug reactions
- Anaphylaxis
- Angioedema
- Food intolerance

Some of the above may be occupational

Category 3 Conditions which are sometimes attributable to external agents but are non-immunological

Examples:

- Irritable bowel syndrome
- Migraine

Category 4 Non-IgE-mediated immunological disease (not the domain of an allergist)

- Contact dermatitis (managed by dermatologists except for drug reactions)
- Extrinsic allergic alveolitis (eg farmer's lung, bird fancier's lung)
- Coeliac disease (gluten enteropathy)

Category 5 Conditions sometimes incorrectly attributed to allergy

Examples:

- Chronic fatigue syndrome
- Symptoms associated with certain psychological disturbances (eg somatisation disorders)
- Hyperventilation syndrome

narrowing and swelling leading to shortness of breath and wheeze. Another pathway involving immune cells known as T helper 2 (Th2) cells is believed to be important in causing chronic allergic disease (continuous blocked nose, on-going wheeziness). This comes about by the release of small proteins called cytokines and chemokines that serve as messengers to recruit other cells into the reaction.

1.3   The common atopic diseases have characteristic symptoms: typically, they include sneezing, wheezing, rashes, swelling, digestive disturbances or collapse. The diagnosis can often be made through careful questioning when obtaining the clinical history. Patients should be asked about the relationship of their symptoms to the time of year (because, for example, tree pollen allergy occurs in spring, and severe asthma that only occurs in August is usually due to allergy to *Alternaria*), their occupation (there are forms of occupational asthma), whether they come into contact with animals (particularly cats, dogs and horses), and whether symptoms occur after food. Enquiries should also be made about dusty and damp living conditions which favour proliferation of the house dust mite. Commonly, several of the common atopic diseases co-exist in the same patient.

1.4 Many patients have symptoms in relation to food. Some have true food allergy, eg to nuts or uncooked fruit or vegetables (particularly children and young adults), but in others there is as yet no evidence that the problem is associated with an alteration in the immune system. For the latter group, the term 'food intolerance' is often used. True food allergy is increasingly common, occurring in over 3% of the population, and can often be recognised by symptoms (typically rash, swelling in the mouth, throat and upper airway and difficulty in breathing) which generally occur within minutes of eating a particular food.

1.5 There are other conditions which are not dependent on IgE where abnormal immune responses to environmental agents again cause the disease. Examples are farmer's lung, certain forms of contact dermatitis and coeliac disease (gluten sensitivity). These are the domain of organ-based specialists and are not dealt with by allergy specialists.

1.6 Box 1.1 lists a further group of disorders where non-specific symptoms occur in the absence of any clear allergic responses to environmental agents. This group includes chronic fatigue syndrome and certain psychological disturbances. Although it is unlikely that there is an allergic basis to these disorders, their undoubted impact on patients and their families needs to be appreciated, and attempts should therefore be made to rule out allergic or other causes. Their management often necessitates a multidisciplinary approach in which allergy specialists may play a role.[1] Unfortunately, the failure of conventional medicine to classify, diagnose and treat these conditions satisfactorily has led to frustration from patients, and to their recourse to many forms of treatment that are as yet unproven.

1.7 A further difficulty in defining allergic diseases is the fact that in some conditions – particularly asthma, chronic nasal symptoms (rhinitis), eczema (dermatitis) and urticaria (itchy skin blotches or hives) – IgE-mediated allergy plays a role in some patients but not in others. For instance, in asthma, allergy may be just one of many triggers of an attack (Fig 1.2); others include virus infections, air pollutions or stress. The importance of the allergy may also change with time, as in eczema and milk/egg allergy, which are much more prevalent in children but are often replaced by other allergies during childhood and adult life.

1.8 Allergic diseases in one form or other affect about one-third of the population, so people are interested in them and they are a popular subject for the media. Allergy is now a separate specialty in the NHS but, although the Royal College of Physicians has approved training programmes and recommended the establishment of more posts, there are still very few consultant physicians and even fewer GPs who have had any formal training in this field. Nevertheless, some NHS allergy clinics have operated for many years, mainly in the larger teaching hospitals. Most were established with academic funding. Many have active research groups attached to them, since there is considerable scientific interest in allergy and allergy-related problems.

1.9 Allergy clinics are often linked to particular specialties, such as chest diseases, ear, nose and throat (ENT) diseases, paediatrics, dermatology and gastroenterology, and are supervised

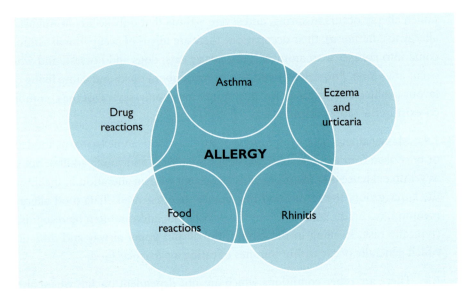

Fig 1.2 **The role of allergy in various diseases.** IgE-mediated allergy plays an important role in some asthmatics for some of the time. In the majority of cases of isolated urticaria, IgE-mediated allergy plays a small role, but urticaria as part of multi-system disease (eg in food, drug, animal allergy or anaphylaxis) is commonly IgE-mediated. Rhinitis (inflammation of the nose) can have both allergic and non-allergic causes. Seasonal allergic rhinitis (hay fever) is entirely due to allergy. In chronic allergic rhinitis, the allergens are usually the house dust mite and animal danders. However, other cases of chronic rhinitis are not IgE-mediated. In food intolerance and in some drug reactions, IgE is not involved.

by a hospital consultant with single-organ specialist qualifications. The changing nature of allergy means that such specialists often receive referrals they are not equipped to diagnose or treat. Furthermore, facilities for allergy testing are limited. A comprehensive and regularly updated list of allergy clinics in the NHS can be obtained from the British Society for Allergy and Clinical Immunology (see Appendix 2).

Reference

1   Bass C, May S. Chronic multiple functional somatic symptoms. *BMJ* 2002;**325**:323–6.

2. The burden of allergic disease in the UK

2.1 Although allergy represents an important cause of patient morbidity and healthcare utilisation, there is little reliable information on the overall disease burden posed by allergic conditions. However, recently the British Society for Allergy and Clinical Immunology (BSACI) commissioned a UK study to determine the prevalence of allergic conditions (excluding occupational allergy), to estimate the healthcare burden posed by these patients, and to assess recent disease trends in the UK population.[1] The key findings of the study are shown in Box 2.1. Full details of the study are provided in Appendix 1.

Box 2.1   Key findings of a UK study on prevalence, healthcare utilisation and recent trends in allergic disorders[1]

▶ Over 18 million people in the UK have at some point been diagnosed as having an allergic illness. Rather more children (40%) than adults (over 30%) have experienced allergy.

▶ In any one year, over 20% of the population (12 million people) have active allergy and are likely to be receiving treatment for it.

▶ Allergic disorders affect all ages, both sexes and all social and ethnic groups in the UK.

▶ International comparisons show that the UK population has the highest prevalence of allergy in Europe and ranks among the highest in the world.

▶ Allergic rhinitis, asthma and eczema are the most commonly experienced expressions of allergy.

▶ Ten per cent of children and adults below their mid-40s (13 million people) have two or more atopic disorders.

▶ Allergy can have a profound impact on quality of life. More than 3% of children are awake at night at least once a week as a result of eczema; twice that number (680,000 children) are woken at least once a week by wheeze.

▶ There were very high growth rates in the prevalence of organ-specific allergic disorders – eczema, asthma, rhinitis – in the latter part of the twentieth century. The upward trends may have ceased for asthma, but the evidence is not definitive. However, it is clear that the disease frequencies of the more serious and systemic allergies, eg anaphylaxis, drug and food allergy, are increasing fast.

▶ Allergic disorders commonly co-exist. Several of the following often occur in the same patient: asthma, rhinitis, eczema, food allergy, drug allergy and anaphylaxis.

▶ Hospital admissions as a consequence of serious anaphylaxis increased seven-fold in the last decade, and admissions for food allergy increased five-fold.

▶ One in 70 children in the UK (160,000 children) are allergic to peanuts, the most common food to cause fatal or near-fatal reactions. The incidence of peanut allergy has trebled in the last four years, although until the 1990s this was a rare disorder.

▶ Allergy costs the NHS an estimated £900 million a year, mostly through prescribed treatments in primary care (10% of the GP prescribing budget), although the cost per case for hospital treatment is considerably higher. This figure does not include the costs of A&E attendances, outpatient consultations and hospital treatment.

▶ Six per cent of GP consultations are for allergic disease.

Reference

1   Gupta R, Sheikh A, Strachan DP, Anderson HR. The burden of allergic disease in the UK. Unpublished study (2002) commissioned by the British Society for Allergy and Clinical Immunology, London.

3. Allergy in children: special issues

3.1   The appropriate treatment of allergy is particularly important in children whose quality of life, education and growth may be greatly affected by their condition. Food allergy is common and can be life threatening – for example peanut allergy now affects 1 in 70 children in the UK. Asthma has been identified as potentially preventable if it is treated in early life. Many children have allergic diseases affecting several organ systems, and are inadequately treated because the allergic trigger(s) goes unrecognised. This chapter sets out the special requirements of children suffering from allergy, and explains why the current deficits in provision are particularly damaging to them.

Prevalence of paediatric allergic diseases in the UK

3.2   Even before the massive increase in prevalence rates for allergic disease, it was estimated that paediatric allergic disease in the USA constituted 28% of all chronic disorders requiring medical attention and resulting in school absence.[1] In the UK, a high percentage of both inpatient and outpatient paediatric workload is related to allergic disease. A recent UK study demonstrated the very high prevalence rates: out of 27,507 children surveyed in 1999, 20.4% were reported to have had asthma in the previous year, 18.2% had had allergic rhinoconjunctivitis, and 16.4% eczema.[2] One or more current atopic symptoms were reported in 47% of all the children. Furthermore, other children had different symptoms that were suggestive of atopic disease, but without a clear-cut diagnosis. These high rates are reflected even in acute paediatric care. In a recent survey of paediatric A&E admissions at St Mary's Hospital, London, 7% of children seen as emergencies were diagnosed as having an allergy disorder.[3] These children required twice the rate of admission and twice the rate of specialist tertiary referral compared to other children attending as emergencies.

Special requirements of children with allergy

Delivery of care

3.3   The Department of Health has emphasised that in the health service children should be seen by health professionals trained in the care of children, in a child-friendly environment. Therefore, if children attend outpatients, they should be seen in a customised children's outpatients; if they are admitted, they should be on a children's day ward or paediatric ward.[4] A National Service Framework (NSF) for children is being established, emphasising the distinct requirements of children.

3.4   In the context of this framework, children with allergy disorders should be managed by paediatric allergy specialists. This is already the case in many other countries which practise medicine to a high standard, including North America and much of Western Europe. Similarly, all staff involved in looking after child patients should be trained in child health; this is particularly important for the nursing staff and dietitians.

3.5   At present in the UK, where there is a severe shortage of paediatricians appropriately trained in allergy, there are circumstances in which adult allergists will have to be involved in the management of children. In all such cases, a named lead paediatrician should also be involved, and this should apply to both outpatient and inpatient practice.

Nutrition, growth and development

3.6   Fundamental to the whole practice of paediatrics is an understanding of growth, development and nutritional requirements. The truism that 'children are not just little adults' is particularly applicable to medicine: the physiology, biochemistry, pharmacology and even anatomy of an infant is fundamentally different to that of an adult. In children, different systems develop at different rates, and without a full understanding of this it is not possible to provide a high standard of medical care. Paediatric care also requires knowledge of children's changing nutritional requirements; a fully trained paediatric dietitian is therefore essential to an effective paediatric allergy service.

Psychological, social and educational issues

3.7   There are complex interactions between organic disease and emotional state, and many allergic disorders cause considerable psychological stress, which can impinge on the child's growth, development, education and career attainments. These difficulties are likely to affect not only the child, but also other family members, particularly parents. For example, children who are allergic to food often develop secondary food phobias, and family members may develop obsessive approaches to the medical issues, for example unnecessary food avoidance. Many children develop needle phobia and then require additional support, particularly if they are to receive immunotherapy.

3.8   Also, allergic disease often leads to disturbed sleep which results in poor concentration, somnolence and impaired cognition. Again, this can have a major impact on education, examination performance and career attainment. Many children with allergic disorders also suffer from bullying and social segregation at school. Children at risk of food-induced anaphylaxis need to avoid the food, and may need to have an adrenaline auto-injector available. Liaison between medical staff and school nurses and teachers/school staff is therefore essential.[5]

Patient education

3.9   As children grow older, their ability to manage their own disease changes. Adolescence represents a transitional period where children are no longer under complete parental control and yet may not be equipped to take on the management of their disease. Patient education should therefore be initiated as early as possible in childhood. Paediatric nurse specialists can educate patients and their families, and liaise with outside agencies to provide a safe environment for the child, where his/her carers and teachers are equipped to manage asthma and anaphylaxis effectively.[5]

Deficits in current paediatric care

Primary care

3.10 Allergic disease comprises a significant percentage of the workload of primary care, and the majority of children with allergy problems – many of whom have multi-organ presentation and appreciable morbidity and mortality – will present first to a GP, and many have their entire care provided by a GP. However, very few GPs have received any training in allergy, so the vast majority of general practices are ill equipped to investigate and manage even straightforward allergic disease (see Chapter 4).

Lack of trained paediatric allergists

3.11 There are less than a handful of NHS paediatric allergists in the UK, which compares badly with countries such as Sweden which has 96 trained paediatric allergy specialists. In Japan, the Paediatric Allergy Society has 2,000 members for a population which is only double that of the UK. The consequence of this severe shortfall is that parents, desperate for treatment for their children, seek help from complementary and alternative medicine. There, children may be subjected to unvalidated testing methods, and are sometimes given potentially dangerous recommendations. For example, it is harmful to put a child on an extensive exclusion diet that has no scientific basis, because of the risk of nutritional compromise and poor growth. The increasing use of so-called 'vaccine treatment' for food allergy is also of concern.

Fragmented specialty care

3.12 As so many children with allergic disease have co-existent eczema, rhinitis, asthma, food allergy etc, they may be seen consecutively in several different settings. Indeed, many go through general paediatrics, ENT, dermatology, chest medicine and gastroenterology clinics. This is a highly inefficient way of delivering healthcare; it also imposes further burdens on the child and family, and causes school absence. Furthermore, the lack of integrated care means that the underlying allergic causes of the different components of allergic disease are often left undiagnosed. Delivery of care for allergic disease by a paediatric allergist would provide a more rational, integrated and cost-effective service.

Medication and side effects

3.13 Fragmented specialty care for children with systemic allergy can also lead to 'steroid loading'. Children may be prescribed topical steroids by the inhaled route, the intranasal route, the cutaneous route and courses of oral steroids for asthma exacerbations, usually with no single specialist taking charge of overall management. This can result in unacceptable side-effects and growth retardation.

3.14 Medication prescribed by those without appropriate training in paediatric allergy can also be dangerous. For example, there is no single dose regimen for medicating children with anaphylaxis, but administration of incorrect doses, eg of injected adrenaline, can have severe consequences. Similar considerations apply to other medications used to treat allergic disease.

Research and preventive measures: the importance of early life events

3.15 Longitudinal birth cohort studies have highlighted that the brunt of allergic disease occurs in early childhood, and much evidence suggests that early life events are critical in programming the individual to develop allergic problems at various stages during life.[6] Indeed, the importance of early life events has been recognised nationally and internationally. In the USA, the National Heart, Lung and Blood Institute at the National Institutes of Health (NIH) has a strategic programme funding research into the early life origins of asthma. The World Allergy Organisation, in collaboration with the World Health Organization (WHO), is currently producing a major document on the prevention of allergy and asthma which focuses extensively on early life.[7] The National Asthma Campaign, in its review of basic asthma research (BARS), has also focused on early life events as an area of particular importance.[8]

3.16 This research could lead to the identification of therapeutic targets that might result in effective primary, secondary and tertiary prevention. There is therefore an urgent need for resources, not only to enhance this research, but also to ensure that there is an appropriate clinical service backing up the research and providing the environment in which preventive strategies can be effectively delivered.

References

1   Mascia AV. Review and assessment of the efficacy of cromolyn sodium, particularly after long-term administration. *Clin Pediatr (Phila)* 1973;**12**:523–4.

2   Austin JB, Kaur B, Anderson HR, Burr M *et al.* Hay fever, eczema and wheeze: a nationwide UK study (ISAAC, international study of asthma and allergies in childhood). *Arch Dis Child* 1999;**81**:225–30.

3   Treffene S, Lack G, Maconochie I. The increasing demand on the National Health Service of allergic conditions within the paediatric population (in preparation).

4   Department of Health. *Welfare of children and young people in hospital.* London: DH, 1991.

5   Vickers DW, Maynard L, Ewan PW. The management of children with potential anaphylactic reactions in the community. *Clin Exp Allergy* 1997;**27**:898–903.

6   Warner JA, Warner JO. Early life events in allergic sensitisation. *BMJ* 2000;**56**:883–93.

7   Johansson SGO, Haahtela T (eds). Prevention of allergy and asthma. Interim Report. *Allergy* 2000;**55**:1069–88.

8   Warner JO. A double-blinded, randomized, placebo-controlled trial of cetirizine in preventing the onset of asthma in children with atopic dermatitis: 18 months' treatment and 18 months' post treatment follow-up. *J Allergy Clin Immunol* 2001;**108**:929–37.

4. Allergy in primary care

4.1   In contrast to many other developed countries, the UK management of allergic disorders takes place almost exclusively within primary care. However, as previously stated, very few primary healthcare professionals have received any formal undergraduate or postgraduate training in the management of allergy. In addition, the specialist services are under-resourced, and poorly distributed.[1]

A UK survey of allergy care in general practice

4.2   A survey of a representative sample of UK GPs, commissioned by the BSACI, was carried out to assess GPs' views on the quality of NHS allergy care, to identify barriers to promoting high-quality care and to establish current training status and needs.[2]

Methods

4.3   A cross-sectional descriptive postal survey of GPs was conducted in May–July 2002 using a self-completed semi-structured questionnaire. Likeert scales (1 to 10) were used to assess GPs' perceptions of allergy services and their own confidence in managing allergic conditions. Binleys Database was used to identify a random sample of 500 GPs from all registered GP principals in the UK.[3] Non-responders ($n = 301$) were followed up with two additional mailings, and a telephone contact over a two-week period immediately after the third mailing.

Results

4.4   Twenty GPs were not contactable because of retirement or ill health. Of 480 eligible GPs mailed, 240 (50%) responded. Respondents had a mean age of 46 years and 137 (57%) were male.

Summary of key findings (Box 4.1)

4.5   More than 80% of GPs thought that NHS allergy services were of poor quality, reflecting deficiencies in both primary and secondary care. The majority of GPs had received no training in the management of allergic disorders, representing the most important barrier to promoting high-quality allergy care within primary care. Only 23% of respondents reported that they were familiar with any guidelines for the management of an allergic condition.

4.6   Almost 80% of GPs rated overall access to a specialist allergist as poor. Of the 240 respondents, 39%, 92% and 25% reported that children in their practices had been diagnosed with multiple food allergies, eczema and dietary/growth problems related to allergies, respectively.

Box 4.1 Key findings of survey on allergy care in general practice[2]

▶ More than 80% of GPs thought NHS allergy services were of poor quality.

▶ Access to specialist services:
  – Very poor provision of specialist referral possibilities was highlighted by the GPs as a primary feature of NHS allergy care.
  – Less than 8% of GP respondents said they had access to a fully comprehensive NHS allergy service.
  – Only one in four of respondents had access to an allergy clinic for their patients.
  – 47% had access to consultants with an interest in allergy (based in dermatology (36%), immunology (28%) and respiratory (16%) departments), but only 17% of them considered the service offered comprehensive.
  – More than half of GPs' referrals to an allergy clinic had to wait more than 100 days.

▶ In primary care:
  – 59% felt the quality of care offered was poor.
  – In general the GPs felt more confident in being able to treat a primary care caseload covering the most common allergies, eg asthma, allergic rhinitis, eczema, anaphylaxis or drug allergy. They felt less confident in managing allergy in children, or food and venom allergy.
  – The main conditions considered for referral were food allergy, eczema, urticaria and anaphylaxis. However, referral was made in less than 25% for most of these conditions.
  – Less than one in four said they were familiar with any guidelines on allergy management, but they had low referral rates even when they were not confident in managing particular allergies.
  – Skin prick tests, which are a simple means of establishing triggers for an allergic reaction, were available in only 4% of the practices sampled.
  – 65% had access to serum-specific IgE tests (RAST). This result in itself indicates ignorance of allergy services since RAST tests are available to all GPs.

▶ Training needs:
  – Half of the GPs sampled had received some training in allergy theory, mostly minimal, at undergraduate level, and not in clinical application. Only 10% of partner GPs, and 17% of practice nurses, had received any clinical allergy training.

RAST = radioallergosorbent test.

Discussion

4.7 The main strength of this survey is the UK-wide sampling frame used and random selection procedure. The results are likely to be generalisable, although the low (50%) response rate was disappointing, suggesting a lack of interest in allergy and that these data may overestimate GPs' knowledge of allergy.

4.8 Over 80% of respondent GPs considered that current allergy service provision throughout the NHS was poor, with deficiencies being most marked in secondary care and in accessing appropriate specialists. In view of the current concerns regarding a severe shortage of allergy specialists/training posts throughout the UK,[1] these results are perhaps unsurprising. Possible barriers to promoting high-quality allergy care within primary care include real or perceived lack of expertise in, and facilities for investigating, allergic conditions. The fact that skin prick test reagents need to be purchased by the GPs without reimbursement of their costs[4] may explain the relatively high proportion of GPs using expensive serum-specific IgE tests.

4.9 The confidence of GPs in managing certain allergies (see Box 4.1) is in contrast to patient opinion obtained from helplines (see Chapter 5), and may reflect a pharmacological approach to treatment rather than an ability to identify an allergic cause and recommend avoidance to the patient, or make a referral to an appropriate specialist.

Further research on primary care

4.10 In addition to the BSACI survey, a recent qualitative study conducted in primary care showed that very few GPs have had any formal training in allergy and even fewer have had clinical exposure in their under- or postgraduate training.[5] Although the data again demonstrate a reasonable degree of self-perceived competence, this is not soundly based and there is much room for improvement.

4.11 Evidence from the helplines run by allergy charities supports this perception of deficiencies in primary care: the majority of helpline callers said they were unable to get allergy advice from their GP. Furthermore, patients with food allergy who subsequently died of anaphylaxis had not been given appropriate advice by their GP, or had been told that 'nothing can be done' about their allergy, or 'just avoid the food' in question (Anaphylaxis Campaign).

4.12 As well as a low level of interest in allergy amongst primary care doctors, the study revealed a fear that getting involved with allergy management would lead to more work in a system that was already overburdened. Many of the GPs surveyed believed that allergy testing was unnecessary and that in most cases treatment and diagnosis were straightforward, with little need for follow-up consultation. Allergy testing was reported to be largely unavailable, and waiting times for specialist referral prohibitively long.

4.13 There was poor knowledge of conventional allergy tests and their interpretation, even though clear dissatisfaction was expressed at allergy tests offered in pharmacies and health food shops. In contrast to the low level of interest expressed by GPs, this study demonstrated that practice nurses were keen to improve care for allergy sufferers, and they expressed a desire to receive training.

Management of allergy in primary care

4.14 Therapy provided in the primary care setting for most of the common allergic diseases (asthma, eczema and rhinitis) is not allergen specific and relies on pharmacotherapy. Although asthma and rhinitis guidelines are underpinned by evidence of the efficacy of aero-allergen avoidance, many primary care practitioners need further convincing of the extent to which diagnostic testing and avoidance measures can effectively, and cost effectively, support their clinical practice. However, it is clear to specialists that accurate identification of the cause, eg a food, drug or animal, is essential and avoidance should play a key part in management. This knowledge urgently needs to be disseminated in primary care.

4.15 One study surveyed attitudes of patients to drug treatment versus allergen avoidance for asthma, and compared this to attitudes of health service professionals.[6] A wide diversity of expectations was found. The majority of patients said they would prefer to be given advice on allergen avoidance rather than rely on drug treatment alone. In primary care, allergen avoidance advice was often given without tests to confirm the diagnosis. By contrast, in secondary care, chest physicians rarely offered allergen avoidance advice.

4.16 The failure to confirm the diagnosis is important. Another study found that when house dust mite avoidance was recommended for patients with asthma in primary care, this was inappropriate in 22% of cases, because the diagnosis was incorrect and had not been confirmed by allergy testing.[7] Allergen avoidance interventions need to be targeted appropriately.

The need for more training

4.17 Improved access to postgraduate training is an essential prerequisite to improving training in primary care. Primary care trusts therefore need to be made aware of the burden of allergic disease and alerted to their responsibilities to provide the resources to meet these needs. Minimum training for those without a special interest in allergy should include an appreciation of the morbidity associated with allergy symptoms and symptom management. For general practices interested in improving their provision of clinical allergy, different models could be employed; for example, the nomination of a lead person, who should receive basic (diploma/degree level) training in allergy and who could manage simple allergy problems and refer on to others.

GP with a special interest (GPSI) in allergy: a new concept

4.18 This is an area of service that does not currently exist. It should not be seen as a cheap alternative to the creation of a high-level allergy service, but rather as an integral part of an overall strategy.

4.19 GPSIs are firmly on the healthcare agenda, the Government having pledged to have 1,000 in post by 2004. A GPSI in allergy or allergy nurse practitioner could manage, within the primary care setting, many of the problems encountered by GPs. Allergy GPSIs should be trained in a dedicated allergy clinic and also undertake appropriate postgraduate training (diploma/degree) in allergy and allergic disorders. As part of their continuing professional development, they should be members of an appropriate professional body such as the British Society for Allergy and Clinical Immunology.

4.20 GPSIs in allergy would play an important role in providing readily accessible expert advice and assessment. They would also provide strategic advice to primary care organisations and other public bodies on issues concerning the management of children and adults with allergic disorders. This should include general written/telephone/email advice to healthcare professionals based in primary care, and also face-to-face consultations with patients referred by members of local primary healthcare teams. These consultations would involve careful history-taking and sometimes necessitate recourse to allergy testing, involving both skin prick testing and *in vitro* serum-specific IgE testing. Some individuals might have other skills such as rhinoscopy and spirometry. S/he would be supported by nurses with specialist allergy training, who would be involved in educating and managing patients. The GPSI should be able to identify much of what is not allergy, referring such cases back to the primary care team for ongoing management.

4.21 Another role for the GPSI must be to raise the level of local knowledge of allergy, identify more severe disease for referral to more specialist care, and have well-developed pathways of communication with the regional consultant allergist and organ-based specialists with an interest in allergy (in ENT, dermatology and respiratory medicine).

Person	Services provided	Skills required	Information/training required
Table 4.1	**Proposed levels of allergy care up to primary care level, and training requirements**		
Patient	Self care	Symptom-specific self-management Symptom control Medicines self-management	Disease-specific information Reputable educational resources Availability of OTC medication Drug-specific information When and where to seek help
Pharmacist	OTC medication Disease-management Referral	Symptom-specific management How to treat allergy with OTC medications	Common allergic symptoms and their presentation Pharmacological management of allergic disease OTC device technique (eg nasal sprays, eye drops) Knowledge of local NHS allergy services: when and where to refer
GP/PN (minimum service to be provided in primary care by GP/PN with no specialist allergy interest)	Allergy symptom management Referral	Symptom management Optimal symptom control using POMs Recognition of severe disease	Common allergic conditions and their manifestations in multiple organ systems Simple algorithms on disease management Availability of diagnostic tests Local availability of NHS allergy services: when and where to refer
Practice lead in allergy (GP/PN with an allergy interest but with no access to increased consultation time or basic diagnostic tests)	Allergy diagnosis Allergy symptom management Referral	History taking Disease management Optimal symptom control using POMs	Epidemiology of allergic disease Genetic influences Environmental influences Current guidelines on disease diagnosis and management Local availability of NHS allergy services: when and where to refer
GP/PN with a special interest in allergy (GP/PN with allergy training with access to increased consultation time and basic diagnostic tests)	Allergy diagnosis Allergy symptom management Simple allergy testing Referral	History taking and interpretation Performance of simple diagnostic tests Interpretation of simple diagnostic tests Identification of allergic triggers Allergen avoidance Rhinoscopy Optimal symptom control using POMs	Epidemiology of allergic disease Genetic influences Environmental influences How to perform and interpret diagnostic tests Allergy and non-allergy: symptoms and management Evidence-based decision-making based on current guidelines on disease diagnosis and management Local availability of NHS allergy services: when and where to refer

GP = general practitioner; PN = practice nurse; OTC = over the counter; POMs = prescription only medicines.

Recommendations

4.22 Recommendations for different types of care up to primary care level are shown in Table 4.1. Proposals for the development of services in primary care and the integration of secondary and tertiary care are given in Chapter 6.

References

1　Ewan PW. Provision of allergy care for optimal outcome in the UK. *Br Med Bull* 2000;**56**:1087–101.

2　Levy ML, Sheikh A, Price D, Zheng X *et al.* A national GP survey of primary care allergy services; current provisions and perceptions of need. Unpublished study (2002) commissioned by the British Society for Allergy and Clinical Immunology, London.

3 Binleys Database. Website: www.binleys.com

4 Sheikh A, Levy M. Costs are a barrier to GPs performing skin prick testing. *Br J Gen Pract* 1999;**49**:67.

5 Cowland N, Whiteside P, Watts R. *Allergy testing communication research.* Unpublished study (2002) prepared for Pharmacia Diagnostics by Insight International. (Personal communication.)

6 McWhirter J, Todd J, Roderick P, Lees S, Warner JO. Patients' and doctors' attitudes to pharmacotherapy versus allergen avoidance in the management of allergic disease. Lifestyles and Asthma Project. AM 10/057 NHS R&D Programme.

7 Sibbald B, Barnes G, Durham SR. Skin prick testing in general practice: a pilot study. *J Adv Nurs* 1997;**26**(3):537–42.

5. The role of allergy charities

5.1   Limitations in UK allergy provision mean that access to expertise and reliable information is often not available to the patient, and independent bodies such as allergy charities therefore have an essential role.

Evidence of need

5.2   The Anaphylaxis Campaign alone receives approximately 20,000 enquiries annually, the vast majority from people seeking information about food allergy. The charity sends out 140,000 leaflets and fact sheets per year, including many bulk orders to schools, education authorities, colleges, hospitals, doctors' surgeries and exhibitions.

5.3   Allergy UK (formerly the British Allergy Foundation) receives 45,000 enquiries annually relating to the wider spectrum of allergy and intolerances, and dispatches 250,000 fact sheets and leaflets per year.

The demand for information

5.4   Allergy charities frequently encounter deep anxiety among families affected by allergies, particularly where those allergies are potentially life-threatening. Lack of information is usually the cause of this distress. It is common for patients to report to allergy charities that they have been unable to obtain adequate help and information from the medical profession; patients' reports of GPs' comments often indicate that the GPs consulted have had minimal training in allergy, or none at all.

5.5   Day-to-day issues, such as confusing food labelling, or the increase in nut traces warnings on food packets, often exacerbate patients' anxieties. Parents of food allergic children talk frequently about 'living with a ticking time bomb', and are unaware that food allergy, whilst sometimes potentially serious, is manageable and that deaths can be prevented.

5.6   Patients may also encounter misleading or inaccurate information on the Internet, in newspapers and magazines and on television and radio, some promoting questionable allergy tests and treatments.

5.7   Outside the family, further demands for information from charities come from schools, restaurants and shops.

Meeting demand

5.8   Registered charities can address this situation by ensuring that in their own information packs and on their websites they provide high-quality, accurate and reliable information, which has been approved by appropriately trained medical experts. Reputable charities should therefore have strong links with the medical and nursing professions.

5.9   Charities can play an equally important role in directing patients towards their nearest NHS allergy services, as GPs and practice nurses are often unaware of the availability of allergy services in their area, despite being sent the BSACI handbook of *National Health Service allergy clinics* (see Appendix 2 for details).

5.10   There are private allergy clinics where practitioners offer 'alternative' approaches and use unvalidated tests (see Chapter 9). Charities can warn patients that advice based on such testing should be viewed with great caution.

5.11   Box 5.1 shows the range of functions currently provided by charities. For a list of UK allergy charities, see Appendix 2.

Box 5.1   Services and information provided by allergy charities

- Patient information via telephone helplines, information packs, videos and websites
- Education and information for schools, colleges, playgroups, youth groups and other lay organisations
- Information and guidelines for the food and catering industries
- Liaison with the medical and nursing professions to provide education and training
- Workshops for teenagers and children with allergies and for parents of allergic children
- Advice and guidance for the Government relating to issues such as food labelling and shortfalls in health provision
- Advice and guidance for local authorities relating to health needs in schools
- Information that highlights areas for research and funding where appropriate
- Information for the media

6. Proposals to improve NHS allergy services

6.1 A previous report by the Royal College of Physicians outlined good allergy practice in 1994,[1] but since then the prevalence of serious allergic disease has increased dramatically: at present, 12 million people (one-fifth of the population) are likely to be receiving treatment for allergy in any one year. This represents a major public health problem.[2] The needs of the UK population and lack of provision of NHS services have already been highlighted.[3] A recent review by the Scottish Executive also emphasised the urgent need for consultant allergists:[4] there are none in Scotland or Wales.

Disorders managed by an allergist

6.2 An allergist deals with a wide range of disorders that cross the organ-based disciplines within medicine. The disorders include: hay fever; perennial rhinitis; allergic eye disease; asthma; occupational asthma; certain skin disorders including angioedema, urticaria and atopic eczema; food allergy; latex allergy; adverse reactions to drugs; allergic reactions to stinging insects; and anaphylaxis. These disorders often co-exist so that allergy presents with multi-system disease. The expertise of an allergist is therefore unique, and distinct from that of organ-based specialists and immunologists. Allergists also have an important role in excluding allergy as a cause of non-specific symptoms.

Lack of expertise and lack of training in allergy

6.3 Despite the high and increasing prevalence of allergic disease, and the recognition of allergy as an NHS full medical specialty, allergy services within the UK are grossly inadequate (Fig 6.1). There is effectively no skill base for allergy management in UK primary care. There are few consultants and few trainees; only six centres in the whole of the UK offer a full-time specialist service. There is no consultant allergist north of Manchester or west of Bournemouth. Currently, most allergy is dealt with by doctors who have little or no training in allergy (ie GPs and consultants in other specialties).

Hospital care: mostly provided by non-allergists

6.4 Much of allergy is treated by organ-based specialists, including chest physicians, ENT specialists, dermatologists, and more recently by immunologists and paediatricians. The majority have had no formal training in allergy and, because their training tends to be in a restricted area, it does not provide the multidisciplinary approach necessary to manage patients with allergies. Many patients have co-existent asthma, eczema, food and drug allergy etc and are referred consecutively to different specialists. This is an inefficient way of delivering healthcare. Furthermore, the underlying allergic causes of the different components often remain undiagnosed. Whilst these specialists have an important role in the management of allergic disorders, a partnership needs to be developed with specialist allergists. Current provision fails to meet standards of clinical governance; the lack of care leads to morbidity, mortality and substantial cost to the NHS (see paragraphs 6.9–6.14), much of which is avoidable.

Allergy care – an investment for life?

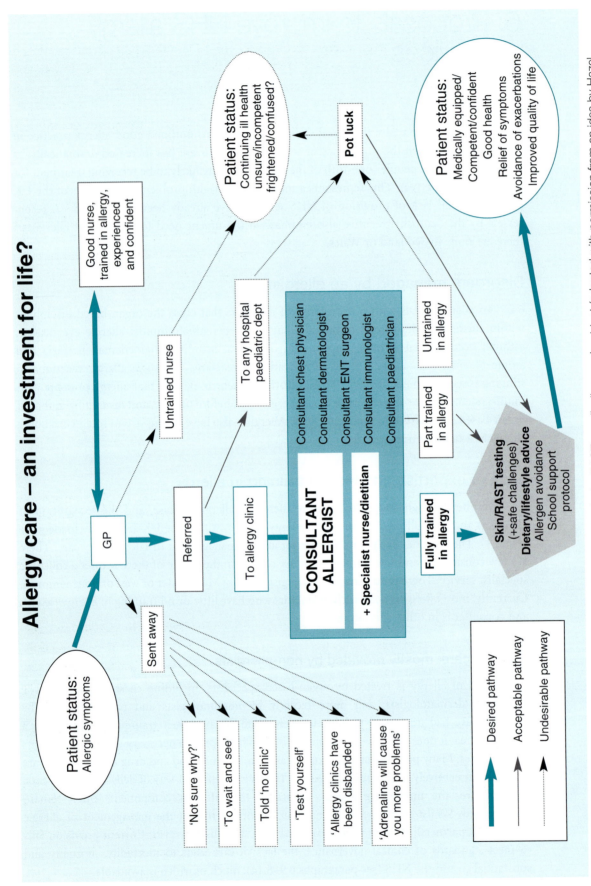

Fig 6.1 Difficulties patients with allergies experience in obtaining help. RAST = radioallergosorbent test (adapted with permission from an idea by Hazel Gowland, Anaphylaxis Campaign).

Multi-system allergy

6.5   Many of the more severe allergic problems do not fall into the remit of an organ-based specialist with an 'interest in allergy'. Problems in this category include life-threatening reactions, eg anaphylaxis during general anaesthesia; venom allergy; severe adverse reactions to drugs; peanut, nut and other food allergies; and latex rubber allergy. These patients should see a consultant allergist in a centre with expertise in these difficult areas with facilities for specialist investigation.

Paediatric allergy

6.6   Allergy commonly occurs in children, but few paediatricians are trained in allergy, leading to inappropriate care and bizarre and poor practice. For example, a child with severe eczema frequently also has food allergy with life-threatening reactions, asthma and rhinitis. Referral to a series of organ-based specialists or a general paediatrician is inappropriate and the allergic aetiology is not usually addressed (Fig 6.1).

Primary care

6.7   If no action is taken, the NHS will continue to leave its staff in primary care responding to the brunt of an allergy epidemic, without the skills or resource base to be able to respond effectively. The service response will continue to be inefficient and ineffective, and patient care will continue to be inadequate.

Helplines

6.8   The difficulty patients have in obtaining advice is evident from the demand for the helplines run by Allergy UK (previously the British Allergy Foundation) and the Anaphylaxis Campaign. These charities provide advice and direct patients to appropriate specialists (see Chapter 5).

Benefits of a specialist allergy service

6.9   The increase in serious allergic disease has driven up the demand for specialist services. There is a need for accurate diagnosis and management, as well as facilities for diagnostic challenge tests, day case services, and allergen immunotherapy (desensitisation) – procedures which should always be carried out in a specialist setting.[5] Identification of the cause of the allergy allows avoidance and amelioration of disease.

6.10   Effective treatment will result in savings to the NHS by reducing A&E attendance and hospital admissions, and will reduce the burden of illness in the allergic patient.[5,6]

6.11   A recent example of cost benefit came from a management strategy for nut allergy which was developed and then evaluated in 567 patients (there was no previous evidence on which to base management). This showed not only a substantial reduction in the number of reactions during follow-up, but also a reduction in their severity: they were mostly mild and readily controlled by self-treatment.[6] Hospital admission and A&E attendance were avoided.

6.12 There is urgent need for information on the best way of diagnosing and managing this type of severe disorder (eg peanut, drug and latex allergy). Production of evidence-based guidelines is an important task for specialists in academic centres, eg management plans for nut allergy and diagnosis of adverse reactions to drugs.[6]

The costs of mismanagement

6.13 Not surprisingly, non-allergists, paediatricians and GPs without training do not know how to manage nut allergy. This leads to inappropriate under- and over-management. Under-management can lead to fatal reactions.[7] Over-management leads to inappropriate provision of medication such as Epipen®, misuse of stretched services, eg community paediatric teams, and anxiety in parents. The debate about the need for auto-injectable adrenaline Epipen® reveals misconceptions and the failure to understand that the use of adrenaline is only part of a complete management strategy.[8,9] Identification of the cause of reactions, expert advice on avoidance, and training in the use of emergency medicines for self-use are essential.[6] A recent study by non-allergists played down the importance of severe and fatal reactions to foods in children[10] but was methodologically flawed, thus underestimating the problem and revealing lack of understanding of allergic problems.[11]

6.14 The cost of failure to refer to an allergist is illustrated by a patient with severe uncontrollable hay fever.[12] His GP resorted to annual injections of a deposteroid, which led to bilateral avascular necrosis of the hip, with the result that the patient, aged 39, was crippled and faces (multiple) bilateral hip replacements. He was subsequently referred to an allergist, desensitised, and his disease was controlled. The efficacy of grass pollen desensitisation (immunotherapy) is well established,[5] but this can only be done in a specialist centre.

Current NHS allergy clinics

6.15 The British Society for Allergy and Clinical Immunology (BSACI), and the British Allergy Foundation (BAF) compiled a list of National Health Service allergy clinics which were NHS consultant-led and based at NHS hospitals throughout the UK (see Fig 6.2). The BSACI handbook of *National Health Service Allergy Clinics* (2001)[13] lists 86 such clinics, and two nurse-led services run by BSACI members (for BSACI details see Appendix 2). There were an additional 15 clinics run by NHS consultants (who were non-BSACI members) identified by BAF. However, only six of these 101 clinics offer services led by a whole-time specialist allergist (Table 6.1). These are based in London (Guy's Hospital, Royal Brompton Hospital and St Mary's Hospital), Cambridge, Southampton and Leicester. These centres have expertise in all types of allergic disease, including the complex problems, and provide a comprehensive

Table 6.1 Allergy clinics in the UK		
Full-time service run by specialists	Part-time service run by specialists	Part-time service offered by consultants in other specialties*
6	9	86

*Consultants with 'an interest' in allergy, usually without formal training in allergy.

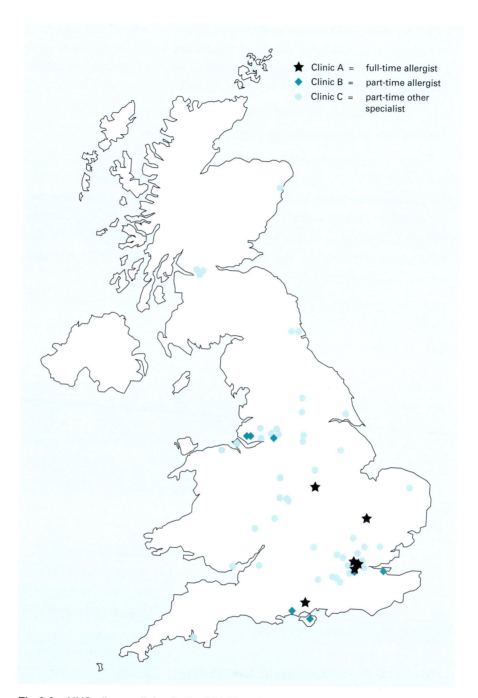

Fig 6.2 NHS allergy clinics in the UK. The distribution of NHS allergy clinics according to the nature of the service provided: (A) full-time services in all types of allergy provided by consultant allergists; (B) part-time services provided by consultant allergists; and (C) part-time services usually in limited areas of allergic disease (eg eczema/urticaria for a dermatologist) provided by consultants in other specialties.

high-quality allergy service with a multidisciplinary approach. In addition, they have an international reputation for research in allergic disease. Five of these six centres (all except Leicester) were developed as academic units with university funding – another indication of the lack of tradition within the NHS of supporting allergy.

6.16 Nine of the 101 clinics are run by a part-time consultant NHS allergist, providing one or two allergy clinic sessions per week. The remaining 86 clinics are run by organ-based or other NHS consultants (for example, in dermatology, asthma, paediatrics or immunology), most of whom offer a limited spectrum of diagnostic and treatment facilities for allergy.

6.17 Table 6.2 shows a list of NHS allergy clinics run by:

(A) full-time allergists (more than five clinics per week)

(B) part-time allergists (one to two clinics per week, arbitrarily assigned a figure of a 0.3 whole-time equivalent (WTE) NHS allergist-led service)

(C) clinics led by organ-based specialists with an interest in allergy offering a limited service (arbitrarily assigned a 0.1 WTE NHS allergist-led service).

These figures are given for the NHS Regions (as defined from 1 April 1999) with populations for comparison. Using the above arbitrary definitions, the WTE NHS allergy specialist-led services are also given.

6.18 The 15 additional part-time clinics run by organ-based specialists (who are not BSACI members and therefore not in the BSACI handbook) equate to 1.5 WTE clinics.

6.19 This comprehensive survey shows that, for the UK population of about 60 million, there is an equivalent of 17.3 (15.8 + 1.5) WTE NHS consultant allergist-led clinics available. This represents one WTE allergist-led clinic per 3.4 million UK population. This is in contrast to one consultant per 100,000 UK population for consultant cardiologists, chest physicians, gastroenterologists, etc (Table 6.3). Even more importantly, there are only six allergy clinics in the UK offering a full-time comprehensive multidisciplinary service and with expertise in complex areas of allergy – a totally inadequate provision. The uneven geographical distribution of allergy clinics is shown in Fig. 6.2.

Demand for services

6.20 Demand is enormous, and waiting lists are high. In Cambridge, the number of patients seen increased by 440% between 1993 and 2000, and simultaneously there has been a change in case-mix to increased numbers of severe cases. Despite the increased workload, referral rate rises inexorably and waiting lists remain unacceptably high for serious disease. This pattern is repeated in all six specialist centres.

Regional commissioning for allergy

6.21 Allergy is one of the specialties on the list for regional commissioning.[14] This means that specified disorders should be dealt with in regional allergy centres where appropriate expertise exists. This recommendation now needs to be implemented. However, the experience from other specialties is that implementation is difficult because of funding pressures, now exacerbated by organisational change and delegation of responsibility to primary care trusts. A central directive is needed to pump-prime these developments. Unless this happens, unnecessary morbidity, mortality and cost to the NHS will continue.

Table 6.2   NHS allergy clinics in the UK: provision of services by region, population and specialist input

Region	Population (millions)	Full-time NHS consultant allergist-led clinics[a] (A)	Part-time NHS consultant allergist-led clinics[a] (B)	Part-time NHS organ-based consultant-led clinics[b] (C)	Total WTE-NHS allergist-led clinics[c] (A+B+C)	Total WTE-clinics led by allergy specialist (A+B)
Northern and Yorkshire	6.3	0	0	7	0.7	0
North West	6.6	0	3	10	1.9	0.9
Trent	5.1	1	0	6	1.6	1.0
West Midlands	5.3	0	0	5	0.5	0
Eastern	5.4	1	0	4	1.4	1.0
South West	4.9	0	0	3	0.3	0
South East	8.6	1	4	10	3.2	2.2
London	7.2	3	2	13	4.0	3.6
Scotland	5.1	0	0	7	0.7	0
Wales	2.9	0	0	4	0.4	0
Northern Ireland	1.7	0	0	2	0.2	0
Total UK	**59.1**	**6**	**9**	**71**	**15.8**	**8.7**

Data from BSACI handbook of *National Health Service Allergy Clinics*, 2001/2002.

Regions: as defined in 1999–2001.

[a] Clinics led by consultant allergists (specialists).

[b] Clinics led by consultants in other specialities who have 'an interest' in allergy, usually without formal training in allergy. These may be held weekly; sometimes within another specialty clinic, ie not in a dedicated allergy clinic; often only offering a service in a restricted area of allergy relating to their own speciality, eg asthma/rhinitis for a respiratory physician, dermatological allergy for a dermatologist, rhinitis for an ENT specialist. Many of these have been set up recently in response to patient demand. Problems arise as patients are referred with problems outwith the consultant's expertise.

[c] Calculated as follows: B counted as 0.3 WTE allergist-led clinic; C counted as 0.1 WTE allergist-led clinic.

WTE = whole time equivalent.

Table 6.3   Provision of allergy services compared to other specialties

Allergy clinics (WTE)[a]	Allergists	Gastroenterologists/cardiologists/ respiratory physicians[b]
1 per 3.4 million population	1 per 2 million population	1 consultant per 100,000 population[b]

[a] Calculated from data on Table 6.2 (this is a composite figure including consultant allergists and consultants in other specialties providing an allergy service) and paragraphs 6.18–6.19.

[b] Data provided by the Royal College of Physicians.

Recommendations

General recommendations for an improved allergy service

1 The provision of allergy care in the NHS must be led by allergy specialists so that appropriate standards of care can be achieved and maintained. Given the scale of what amounts to a national epidemic, the front line for allergy management must be within primary care. However, with virtually no primary care skill base to work from, clinical leadership must come initially from specialist centres. They will need to take on the dual role of diagnosis and management of the most complex cases, and of supporting the development of capacity within primary care.

2 The NHS therefore needs to move forward on two fronts. As an essential first step, more consultant posts and funded training posts in allergy are required. These must become the core leadership for a national training and clinical development initiative for the whole service. They must also provide the essence of a genuinely national allergy service for the NHS. The creation of these posts, and their appropriate service development context, requires recognition of the need for them by the Department of Health, the Workforce Numbers Advisory Board (WNAB), primary care trusts, regional commissioners and trust managers.

3 The report therefore proposes the setting up of appropriately staffed regional allergy centres geographically distributed across the whole country. Based on the service models which exist in those parts of the UK fortunate enough to have established specialist centres, they will give equality of access to appropriate allergy services for adults and children in all parts of the country. They will also provide expertise and lead the development of other local services, networking with organ-based specialists and GPs (Fig 6.3).

4 Regional commissioning for specialist allergy must also be implemented. This will require central direction.

The specific recommendations of the report are grouped below under five headings.

Specific recommendations

Regional allergy centres

5 The working party endorses the recommendations of the BSACI that each of the eight NHS Regions in England (as configured in 2001, each with a population of approximately 5–7 million), as well as Scotland, Wales and Northern Ireland, should have an absolute minimum of one regional specialist allergy centre.[15]

6 Staffing levels required to set up a new centre or develop an existing one are as follows:

▶ a minimum of two new/additional (WTE) consultant allergists (for adult services) offering a multidisciplinary approach. This is the minimum requirement to provide necessary cover for diagnostic procedures and specialist treatment.

▶ a minimum of two full-time allergy nurse specialists

▶ one half-time adult dietitian and one half-time paediatric dietitian with specialist training in food allergy

▶ two consultants in paediatric allergy, supported by paediatric nurse specialists and dietitians with expertise in paediatric allergy

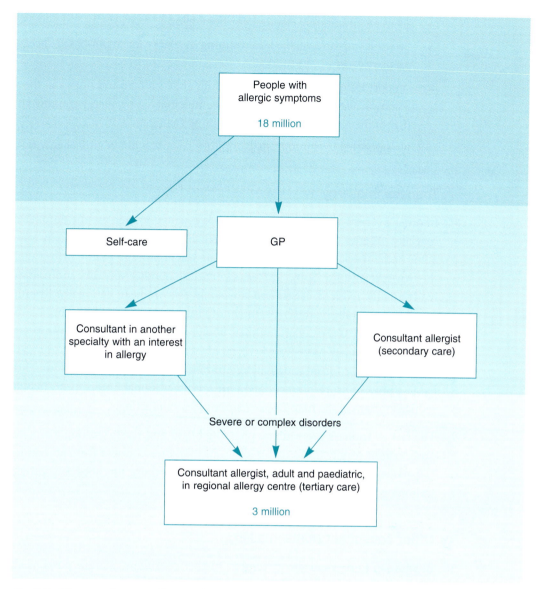

Fig 6.3 Proposed care pathways for patients with allergy. Numbers shown in green are approximate.

> facilities for training for two specialist registrars in allergy (in some centres).

Importantly, this would provide an even geographical distribution of specialist allergy services throughout the UK.

7   The regional centres should:

> provide specialist expertise for difficult allergic disease throughout their Region (tertiary care), including allergic disorders recognised for regional commissioning[14]

> care for allergic disease in the local population which cannot be dealt with in general practice (secondary care)

> deal with adults and children (adult and paediatric services might be offered from the same unit, with communal infrastructure, depending on local circumstances)

> ▶ act as an educational resource for the Region

> ▶ network with and enable local training in allergy for organ-based specialists and paediatricians

> ▶ support training at local level for family practitioners and nurses in the management of common allergies in primary care (complemented by allergy training courses, such as that of the National Respiratory Training Centre)

> ▶ be supported by appropriate laboratory resources for *in vitro* allergy testing.

Trainees in allergy

8 In order to create new consultant posts it is essential to increase the number of trainees in the specialty. Allergy was disadvantaged when the Calman training system was introduced: the name of the specialty was changed and there was an interim period before allergy was added to the new specialist list. Some trainees switched to another specialty and training numbers were inadvertently reduced. There are now only five trainees nationally. Training numbers are controlled centrally by the Department of Health and the WNAB according to a mathematical formula, linked to consultant numbers and growth. The rules are inappropriate and need to be relaxed for a small specialty where rapid expansion (and hence an increase in trainees) is needed. The case for increased allergy trainees was put to the WNAB in 2001 and 2002. This led to a provisional recommendation for seven additional funded posts in 2003/05, which was reduced to zero at the final Department of Health meeting.

9 The lack of trainees is creating a planning blight and trusts wishing to create new consultant posts cannot readily find suitable applicants, and recruitment from abroad has occurred. The Department of Health and the WNAB must recognise the need and provide more funded training posts in allergy.

Other consultant posts in allergy

10 In addition to regional allergy centres, further consultant allergist posts need to be created in other teaching hospitals and district general hospitals in each Region to deal with local needs (numbers have been calculated).[16] One model might be for a shared appointment between trusts. This is a longer-term aim and should follow the establishment of regional centres.

Training in allergy for primary care

11 Primary care must ultimately provide the front line care in NHS management of allergy, as for most other healthcare, but considerable development is needed if it is to provide care that is clinically appropriate for a twenty-first century health service.

12 The training of GPs and practice nurses in allergy needs to be improved. There are currently a number of allergy courses for GPs and practice nurses, eg through the National Respiratory Training Centre or Southampton University School of Medicine, or one-day training courses in different parts of the country run by the BSACI. However, a much more comprehensive nationwide approach is needed, covering primary care training across the NHS.

Organ-based specialists with an interest in allergy

13 Networking with specialist centres should improve allergy services. Organ-based specialists will continue to contribute to allergy care and have primary responsibility for patients with asthma and eczema, in patients with single-organ involvement. They should network with the specialist allergist who can act as a resource in identifying/managing allergy.

Mechanisms for expansion

The devolution of finance and purchasing of services to primary care trusts (PCTs) means that it is difficult to set up new initiatives, because of fierce competition for resources with established specialties. In Regions with a non-existent service (much of the UK), allergy lacks a voice. Allergy is often confused with immunology and not understood by PCTs or regional commissioners.

▶ A central directive is required to develop allergy services. National Service Frameworks (NSFs) have been a way of developing services but at present it is not possible to set up a new NSF. Discussions have been held with the Health Minister and senior officials at the Department of Health with responsibility for allergy.

▶ The addition of allergy services to the regional commissioning list is an important step forward.[14] This means those responsible for regional commissioning should recognise the necessity for specialist allergy services. In a region with commissioning of services, a model set-up could be developed and adopted in other areas, particularly those with no local expertise. The cost of setting up regional centres with two new consultants and support staff for adult services would be approximately £350,000 per annum per Region (with one trainee) or £3.85 million per annum for the UK. The cost for England would be £2.8 million. Since there are not enough trainees available, the development would be gradual, at a lower annual cost. The cost would double to provide paediatric allergy services. There would be substantial savings, in reduced hospital admissions, A&E attendance, drug costs etc, and reduced morbidity and mortality.

▶ The inadequacy of services should be highlighted by patient support groups.

References

1   Royal College of Physicians and Royal College of Pathologists. *Good allergy practice: standards of care for providers and purchasers of allergy services within the National Health Service.* London: RCP, 1994.

2   International Study of Asthma and Allergies in Childhood (ISAAC). Worldwide variation in prevalence of symptoms of asthma, allergic rhinoconjunctivitis, and atopic eczema. *Lancet* 1998;351:1225–32.

3   Ewan PW. Provision of allergy care for optimal outcome in the UK. In: Kay AB (ed) Allergy and allergic diseases: with a view to the future. *Br Med Bull* 2000;56:1087–101.

4   *Immunology and allergy services in Scotland.* Edinburgh: Scottish Medical and Scientific Advisory Committee, Scottish Executive, 2000.

5   Durham SR, Walker SM, Varga E-M, Jacobson MR *et al.* Long term clinical efficacy of grass-pollen immunotherapy. *N Engl J Med* 1999;341:468–75.

6   Ewan PW, Clark A.T. Long-term prospective observational study of patients with peanut and nut allergy after participation in a management plan. *Lancet* 2001;351:111–15.

7   Bock SA, Munoz-Furlong, Sampson HA. Fatalities due to anaphylactic reactions to foods. *J Allergy Clin Immunol* 2001;107:191–3.

8   Unsworth J. Adrenaline syringes are vastly overprescribed. *Arch Dis Child* 2001;**84**:410–11.

9   Ewan PW, Clark AT. Prescribing epinephrine alone is not the complete answer to managing food allergy. *Arch Dis Child* 2002; letter.

10 Macdougall CF, Cant AJ, Colver AF. How dangerous is food allergy in childhood? The incidence of severe and fatal reactions across the UK and Ireland. *Arch Dis Child* 2002;**86**:236–9.

11 Clark AT, Ewan PW. Food allergy in childhood: have the dangers been underestimated? *Arch Dis Child* 2003;**88**:79–81.

12 Nasser SMS, Ewan PW. Depot corticosteroid causing avasular necrosis of both hips in hayfever – is this treatment still appropriate? *BMJ* 2001;**322**:1589–91.

13 British Society for Allergy and Clinical Immunology. *National Health Service Allergy Clinics,* 3rd edn (2001-2002). London: BSACI, 2001.

14 Department of Health. *National specialised services definitions set.* Specialist services for allergy definition no 17 (all ages). DH website: www.doh.gov.uk

15 Ewan PW, Durham SR. NHS Allergy services in the UK: proposals to improve allergy care. *Clin Med* 2002;**2**:122–7.

16 Royal College of Physicians. Allergy. In: *Consultant physicians working for patients: the duties, responsibilities and practice of physicians,* 2nd edn. London: RCP, 2001:45–53.

PART TWO

Allergy: a brief guide to causes, diagnosis and management

7. Environmental exposure to airborne allergens

Environmental aerobiology considers any airborne biological particles, such as dander from animals, bioaerosols, material from excreta, bacteria and viruses, fungal spores and pollen, and is concerned with both indoor and outdoor locations.

Sources of outdoor inhaled allergens

The National Pollen Monitoring Network provides information on the timing of pollen and spore seasons, regional differences and trends in aero-allergen concentrations in the ambient atmosphere. The UK has one of the most comprehensive pollen monitoring networks in the world: 33 monitoring sites work with common methodology and quality control to produce standardised data, stored in a central databank at the National Pollen Research Unit, University College Worcester.

Notable differences occur regionally in the timing and severity of pollen seasons. Also, the pollen seasons for many spring-flowering trees have become earlier, and evidence shows a recent trend towards more severe grass pollen seasons in many areas. Pollen allergens can be present on very small suspended particles and aerosols, and can be altered by air pollutants.

Allergenic pollen and spores in the UK and seasonal variation

Many types of allergenic pollen occur in the UK (see Fig. 7.1, overleaf). Grass pollen is by far the most important, as about 95% of hay fever sufferers are allergic to this. The grasses have evolved comparatively recently and are all closely related, giving a high degree of overlap. Most of the pollen emanates from only 10 species, due to their widespread distribution and high pollen productivity. Collectively, these have a main flowering season from late May until the start of August with two peaks, one in June and the other in July.[1] In the peak months of June and July, grass pollen concentrations are highest on warm dry days with a gentle wind; within this type of day there are typically two peaks, in the morning and late afternoon. Grass pollen counts are low when the weather is cool and blustery and the pollen is washed from the air by rain.

The second most important allergenic pollen type is birch pollen (approximately 25% of hay fever sufferers are allergic to birch). The birches have a main pollen season during April and May, and cross-react with many other members of the birch family including alder and hazel, which flower earlier in the spring, and hornbeam, which flowers later. There are also cross-reactions with certain foods, most notably apples, kiwi and stoned soft fruits, as well as raw vegetables (eg celery, avocado, potato). This allergic 'cross-reactivity' with birch pollen is attributed to a group of storage proteins (profilins) that also occurs in uncooked fruit and vegetables.

Other trees have allergenic pollen, but the pollen seasons for late spring- and summer-flowering trees overlap with that for grass and therefore their importance has been masked.

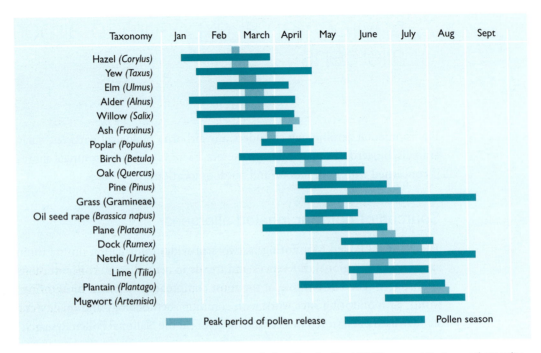

Fig 7.1   Pollen calendar showing the general situation in the UK. The exact timing and severity of pollen seasons will differ from year to year, depending on the weather, and also regionally, depending on geographical location. (Information supplied by the National Pollen Research Unit, University College Worcester.)

In the UK, very little information is available about sensitivity to weed pollen. The main types are nettle (with some closely related but more allergenic *Parietaria* in south and central UK), plantain, dock and goosefoot. The peak pollen seasons for all of these are in late summer and early autumn.

Very few people are truly allergic to pollen from crops such as oil seed rape; reported 'allergic' reactions in the vicinity of the flowering crops are largely attributed to the irritant effects of volatile organic chemicals that are emitted from the plants.

The numbers and types of fungal spores in the air differ with season, geographical location, vegetation, land use, weather and time of day. Some spores are released during warm dry weather, whereas others require mechanical release by rain splash, or need high relative humidity. The most widespread are *Cladosporium* and *Alternaria* which, although found throughout the year, peak in late summer during harvesting and are an important cause of severe asthma. *Aspergillus* and *Penicillium* are also widespread generally. Overall peak concentrations of spores occur in early autumn.

Potentially the duration of exposure to allergenic pollen and spores in the ambient air could be from January through to October, depending on weather conditions and sensitivity, with the peak occurring in June and July. Many people do not know which pollen or spore types they are allergic to. For sufferers who are sensitive to a wide variety of plant pollens, symptoms can extend over many months.

Temporal differences and trends

The sequence of the seasons for the various pollen and spore types follows a set pattern but considerable differences occur annually in the timing and severity of the seasons, due to weather. Over the last few decades, the trend towards climatic warming has resulted in the timing of pollen seasons for many trees becoming earlier.[2] For those who are allergic to tree and grass pollen, the earlier start of pollen release means an extension of the 'allergy' season.

Regional contrasts

Within the UK, some of the differences in the length and severity of pollen seasons are reflected in the prevalence of hay fever and pollen-related asthma.

Pollen seasons differ geographically over the UK because of contrasts in local climate, vegetation and topography. In addition to these natural variables, differences in agriculture and land use exert influences on the spectrum and abundance of pollen and spores. At the regional level, notable contrasts exist depending on latitude and distance from the coasts. The most severe grass pollen seasons typically occur in the midlands, due to the local vegetation and central position.

Differences in pollen concentrations between urban and rural areas can be very marked. In moderate-sized towns, the concentrations of grass pollen are typically 50% lower than in the surrounding countryside. On the other hand, the concentrations of allergenic tree pollen can be at least as high.

Pollen allergens and pollution

Research indicates that some pollen allergen can be transferred by physical contact to particles including diesel exhaust. In addition, grains can burst by osmotic shock during thunderstorms and heavy rainfall to release small starch granules (~2.5 µm) containing the allergens. This fraction has been implicated in thunderstorm asthma.[3] Air pollutants also have effects on pollen allergens, eg exposure to ozone can lead to increased allergen release.[4]

Avoidance measures

It is impossible to avoid contact with pollen entirely but some sensible avoidance measures can be taken, reducing exposure both outdoors and indoors. Knowledge of allergen seasons will also allow for early introduction of prophylactic medication and better control of the disease.

Sources of Indoor inhaled allergens

The indoor environment of modern homes contains many substances that can induce allergic sensitisation and aggravate allergic disease in susceptible individuals. The major biological sources of allergens range from mites, insects (eg cockroaches), animals (cats, dogs and rodents) and fungi, to pollens derived from outside.

House dust mites (Fig 7.2, overleaf)

In 1964, Voorhorst suggested that allergen from dust mites was the main house dust allergen, contradicting the previous idea that the dust allergen was produced just by a chemical reaction.

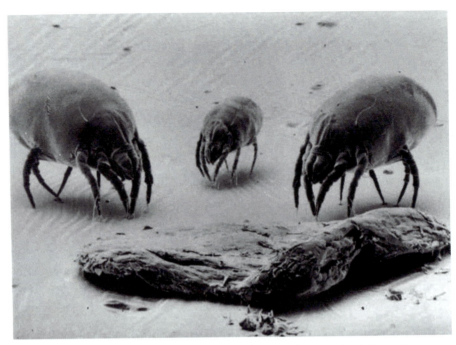

Fig 7.2   House dust mites. Allergy to dust mites is an important risk factor for rhinitis, asthma and eczema in the UK.

This marked the beginning of extensive research into the relationship between dust mites and allergy, and into ways to reduce mite allergen exposure. Analysis of dust samples from homes in different parts of the world shows that many mite species occur in household dust. Dust mites belong to the same class as spiders, scorpions and ticks. They feed on human skin scales, fungi, bacteria and various types of organic waste. In order to digest food, mites produce a number of enzymes, which accumulate in large amounts in their faeces and are a potent cause of allergy in humans.

Mites are found in the high-use areas of the home, such as beds, carpets and upholstered furniture. High humidity is essential for their survival. The sealing of homes to prevent draughts and heat loss, the increase in soft furnishing and carpets, and reduced ventilation of modern homes is contributing to rising dust mite exposure. Mite abundance does not appear to be affected by vacuum cleaning, and well-maintained homes may still contain a large number of mites.

Dust mites are a major cause of allergy. Allergy to dust mites is associated with hay-fever-like symptoms throughout the year (perennial allergic rhinitis) and asthma, and it is likely that exposure to mite allergens exacerbates eczema symptoms in some adults and children.

Measures to reduce exposure to mites[5]

There are a variety of measures that can be used to reduce exposure, including the use of bedding covers that are impermeable to mite allergens. These measures make an important contribution to treatment, in appropriate patients where the diagnosis has been established. Providing such advice is an important role of an allergy service.

Domestic pets

Domestic animals are the second largest source of indoor allergens in the UK. The most common household pets are cats and dogs, with about 15 million registered cats and dogs in UK homes. Surprisingly, many people who are sensitive to pet allergens still choose to keep pets in their homes. Allergic reactions to cats, dogs and horses occur frequently, and sensitisation to one animal is often accompanied by sensitisation to other related or non-related species. Animal allergens are also potential occupational sensitisers for laboratory staff who work with animals (especially mice and rats), and for veterinarians.

Exposure to allergens of domestic pets occurs not only in homes with animals, but also in homes that have never housed a pet, and in public places where allergens have been transported on the clothing of pet owners. This suggests that individuals living in homes without an animal can be exposed to low levels of pet allergens in their homes, and that 'passive' exposure could contribute to symptoms in pet allergic patients. Indoor air pollutants, especially passive exposure to tobacco smoke, have also been shown to enhance sensitisation to indoor allergens.

Pet ownership, sensitisation and allergic disease

The effect of pet ownership in early life on the subsequent development of allergen sensitisation and atopic disease is an area of controversy. Some studies found that exposure to cats and dogs in early life caused allergic sensitisation later in childhood.[6] However, others found a protective effect, but only if the cat is present from the start of the child's life.[7,8] There are two possible explanations for these apparently contradictory findings. Cat allergen is found everywhere and passive exposure of non-pet-owners outside the domestic environment may lead to allergy. However, pet owners exposed to very high levels of allergen in early life may initially mount an allergic response, which may later be replaced by a form of tolerance.[9] Alternatively, exposure of young children to high levels of bacterial products in homes with pets may be protective. Either way, pet allergic patients who experience symptoms upon exposure should make every attempt to reduce the amount of allergen to which they are exposed.

Pet allergen avoidance[5]

The only way to substantially reduce the exposure level to cat or dog allergen is not to have one in the home. However, even after permanent removal of an animal from a home it can take many months for the allergen reservoir levels to fall. A large number of pet allergic individuals will continue to live with their animal and control of allergen levels may be attempted in a variety of ways, although usually with little effect.

Indoor fungi

Fungi and their spores are found whenever there is an opportunity for organic matter to decay. Moulds such as *Aspergillus* and *Penicillium* are troublesome indoors, especially when there are damp conditions. Reduced exposure occurs if rooms are dry and well ventilated. Outdoor moulds such as *Cladosporium* and *Alternaria* have been linked to worsening asthma in allergic individuals.

References

1   Emberlin JC. Grass tree and weed pollens. In Kay AB (ed) *Allergy and allergic diseases.* Oxford: Blackwell Science, 1997:835–8.

2   Emberlin J, Mullins J, Corden J, Millington W *et al.* The trend to earlier Birch pollen seasons in the UK: A biotic response to changes in weather conditions ? *Grana* 1997;**36**:29–33.

3   Newson R, Strachan D, Archibald E, Emberlin J *et al.* 1997 Effect of thunderstorms and airborne grass pollen on the incidence of acute asthma in England, 1990-94. *Thorax* 1997;**52**:680–5.

4   Emberlin J. The effects of air pollution on allergenic pollen. *Eur Respir Rev* 1998; **8**:(53):164–7.

5   Custovic A, Murray CS, Gore RB, Woodcock A. Environmental allergen control. *Ann Allergy Asthma Immunol* 2002;**88**:432–41.

6   Lau S, Illi S, Sommerfeld C, Niggemann B, Bergmann R *et al.* Early exposure to house dust mite and cat allergens and development of childhood asthma: a cohort study. *Lancet* 2000:**356**:1392–7.

7   Hesselmar B, Aberg N, Aberg B, Eriksson B, Bjorksten B. Does early exposure to cat or dog protect against later allergy development? *Clin Exp Allergy* 1999;**29**:611–7.

8   Custovic A, Hallam CL, Simpson BM, Craven M *et al.* Decreased prevalence of sensitisation to cats with high exposure to cat allergen. *J Allergy Clin Immunol* 2001;**108**:537–9.

9   Platts-Mills T, Vaughan J, Squillace S, Woodfolk J, Sporik R. Sensitisation, asthma, and a modified Th2 response in children exposed to cat allergen: a population-based cross-sectional study. *Lancet* 2001;**357**:752–6.

8. Common diseases associated with allergy

Asthma

Asthma is among the most common chronic diseases of the western world, and accounts for much ill-health and time off school and work. It is a condition characterised by episodes of wheezy breathlessness, but in children may cause only cough, particularly at night. The bronchial airways are inflamed and there is also bronchial hyper-responsiveness ('irritable or twitchy airways'). In adults and children, the asthmatic response can be triggered by a wide variety of agents. These include allergens, viral infections, exercise, exposure to fumes and other irritants, certain drugs (beta-blockers, aspirin and other anti-inflammatory agents), food and drink. Allergy is a common cause of childhood asthma, and the substantial increase in incidence of asthma over the last three decades is largely allergy driven.

Asthma which is undertreated can be readily triggered by these various factors (eg allergens or infections), acting either alone or in combination. When considering the cause of acute severe attacks, it is important to establish the relative contribution of ongoing poor asthma control versus triggers, by means of careful history-taking and investigations to establish which allergen(s) are contributory. In cases of episodic acute asthma, the cause is readily identified: for example, a patient with seasonal allergic asthma wheezes when the pollen count is high, has sensitisation to pollen (as revealed by skin prick testing or measurement of allergen-specific IgE), and is symptom-free for the rest of the year. Seasonal allergic asthma can occur alone or in combination with summer hay fever. Allergy may also be an important factor in asthmatics with chronic wheeziness; for example, if they are sensitised to the house dust mite, mould, fungi or allergens from domestic animals. However, due to their non-specific bronchial hyper-responsiveness, such people will almost invariably wheeze after exposure to non-specific triggers, such as smoke and fumes, and may have a prolonged wheezing episode after a viral infection such as the common cold.

Identification of potential allergic triggers is an important aspect of asthma care and leads to improved management and decreased morbidity. The significance of a specific allergen in a particular individual may be suspected from the clinical history. House dust mite allergy is an important trigger in perennial asthma and should be considered if symptoms occur or get worse at night, after vacuuming and bed making, or when the patient stays in old, dusty or damp premises. Asthmatic symptoms related to animal dander are more easily identified and in severe cases can even be provoked by contact with the clothes of someone who has handled or ridden a horse. Exposure to an allergen or sensitising chemical in the workplace must always be considered. Allergy to the moulds *Alternaria* or *Cladosporium* is an important cause of severe seasonal asthma in late summer and autumn. Patients with this type of allergy have recurrent severe asthma at the same time each year, often requiring hospital admission. Yet the allergic trigger usually goes unrecognised, unless the patient is seen by an allergist. Awareness of the cause in this and other allergies allows preventive treatment by avoidance and prophylactic inhaled corticosteroids at the appropriate time. Morbidity is then reduced and cost savings made.

Sometimes the clinical history does not point to the allergen. For instance, many mould spores are allergenic but may be difficult to incriminate because they are so common, particularly in damp and poor housing conditions.

About 25% of asthma is not associated with demonstrable IgE-dependent allergy. These patients are sometimes called 'intrinsic' or 'non-atopic' asthmatics and their disease often starts in later life. A proportion of these late-onset asthmatics have accompanying rhinitis, sinusitis and recurrent nasal polyps. They are frequently intolerant of aspirin and other non-steroidal anti-inflammatory drugs (NSAIDs), and must be identified early in order to prevent the potentially catastrophic consequences of inadvertent ingestion. Many of these aspirin-intolerant asthmatics have co-existent rhinitis and nasal polyps and are frequent attendees at ENT departments undergoing repeated polypectomies. In some cases, 20 or more separate operations have been carried out at annual intervals. This disorder is due to disordered leukotriene metabolism and is unrelated to IgE antibody.[1] It is important to emphasise that this is a severe subtype of asthma which is often very difficult to treat. Awareness of the importance of this condition is paramount in reaching a diagnosis, and such patients complain of severe asthma, requiring maintenance therapy with oral corticosteroids. Intractable cases should be referred to a specialist allergy clinic or a respiratory physician with experience of this condition.[2]

The presence of atopy (specific IgE in the blood or positive skin prick tests to one or more of a range of common aeroallergens) increases the likelihood of developing clinical asthma. Thus, allergy is often a key element in the early stages of the asthmatic disease process. However, if chronic changes in the airways are allowed to become established (airway remodelling), allergy becomes only one of many environmental factors in the typical chronic asthmatic, and other non-allergic factors increase in importance in provoking asthmatic symptoms.[3] It then becomes more difficult to determine what proportion of symptoms are due to specific allergens, even though two-thirds of these patients are atopic.

The precise contribution of the triggers in asthma, including allergy, is of practical importance where the triggers can be easily identified and avoided. Other important potential triggers or precipitating factors are stress and hormonal influences, including menstruation, pregnancy, menopause, and those following childbirth. Acid reflux is also an aggravating factor in asthma. Thus, the twenty-first century evaluation of a patient with asthma involves identification of individual triggers, an assessment of his or her environment, and formulation of a strategy to prevent both acute attacks and progression to the more intractable chronic state. This requires knowledge of allergens and the characteristics of disorders they cause. With the availability of newer, specific treatments for asthma, such as an anti-IgE monoclonal antibody,[4] it becomes even more important to establish the patient's 'asthma-phenotype' in order to predict an individual's treatment response. It is no longer acceptable to ignore the underlying causes and treat all asthmatics as a uniform group, especially when patients themselves wish to know more about the underlying causes for their disease.

Management

Allergen avoidance is important when allergy is a major trigger (as it is in the majority of children and young adults with asthma), and reduces the need for drug therapy.

Guidelines such as the British Thoracic Society asthma guidelines[5] are evidence-based or reflect best practice in relation to drug therapy. Wherever possible, patients should be encouraged to take responsibility for managing their drug regime. In general, patients with mild intermittent symptoms may use short-acting relaxants to relieve wheeze, but anyone with frequent or continuous symptoms should receive regular preventive therapy.

β_2-adrenergic agonist bronchodilators

The most effective drugs for the relief of wheeze are β_2-adrenergic agonists, eg salbutamol and terbutaline. Long-acting beta-adrenergic agonists (salmeterol, formoterol) should not be used as sole agents but are recommended as first choice adjunct therapy to inhaled corticosteroids, as there is evidence of improvement in lung function and fewer exacerbations. β_2-agonists are effective in protecting against exercise-induced asthma. Patients who need a short-acting beta-agonist more than twice daily should be prescribed inhaled corticosteroids for regular use. The bronchodilator is then used as required as 'rescue' medication.

Inhaled corticosteroids

The introduction of inhaled corticosteroids greatly improved asthma control. The dose required should be reviewed periodically to minimise side effects. All inhaled steroids are absorbed into the bloodstream to an extent: newer steroids such as fluticasone and mometasone are almost entirely destroyed in the liver, whereas older steroids such as beclomethasone diproprionate and budesonide are metabolised to a lesser extent.

Leukotriene receptor antagonists

Leukotriene receptor antagonists (LTRAs) are effective in blocking exercise-induced wheeze, and also help in a proportion of people with asthma of all severities, especially those with sensitivity to aspirin and related drugs. They are used as adjunct therapy in patients not controlled by inhaled steroids. More recently, LTRAs have been shown to be active in the treatment of rhinitis.

Other drugs

The role of methyl-xanthines (aminophylline and theophylline) is being re-evaluated. Anti-cholinergic drugs, such as ipratropium bromide and oxitropium, are useful in the treatment of severe asthma. Sodium cromoglycate and nedocromil are now used less, but appear to work best in children.

Immunotherapy

In a number of countries, immunotherapy (desensitisation or hyposensitisation) is increasingly used as a treatment for asthma. It appears to be most effective in younger patients with only a single or few allergic sensitisations and mild to moderate disease, especially when accompanied by allergic rhinitis.[6] In these subjects, immunotherapy may reduce the onset of new allergic sensitisations,[7] and reduce non-specific bronchial hyper-reactivity. However, except in very special circumstances, attempted treatment of the allergic component of asthma by immunotherapy is not recommended in the UK because of an increased risk of anaphylactic bronchconstriction.

References

1   Nasser SMS, Lee TH. Leukotrienes in aspirin-sensitive asthma. In: Szczcklik A, Gryglewski RJ, Vane JR (eds) *Eicosenoids, aspirin and asthma* (Lung Biology in Health and Disease series). New York: M. Dekker, 1998: vol 114; 317–35.

2   Nasser SMS, Lee TH. Aspirin sensitive asthma. In: Holgate S, Busse W (eds) *Inflammatory mechanisms of aspirin-sensitive asthma* (Lung Biology in Health and Disease series). New York: M Dekker, 1998: vol 117, chapter 35; 823–44.

3   Kay AB (ed). *The allergic basis of asthma.* London: Baillière Tindall, 1988.

4   Milgrom H, Fick RB Jr, Su JQ, Reimann JD *et al.* Treatment of allergic asthma with monoclonal anti-IgE antibody. rhuMAb-E25 Study Group. *N Engl J Med* 1999;**341**:1966–73.

5   British Thoracic Society, Scottish Intercollegiate Guidelines Network (SIGN). British guideline on the management of asthma. *Thorax* 2003;**58** (Suppl 1):i1–i194.

6   Abramson MJ, Puy RM, Weiner JM. *Allergen immunotherapy for asthma* (Cochrane review). In: the Cochrane Library, Issue 3. Oxford: Oxford Update Software, 2001.

7   Pajno G, Barbero G, De-Luca F, Morabito L, Parmiani S. Prevention of new sensitisations in asthmatic children monosensitised to house dust mites by specific immunotherapy. *Clin Exp Allergy* 2001;**31**:1392–7.

Allergic rhinitis

Hay fever or seasonal allergic rhinitis refers to the characteristic symptoms of nasal itch/sneezing, watery nasal discharge and congestion, which occur in sensitised individuals during seasonal pollen exposure and are often accompanied by allergic eye symptoms. Although frequently trivialised, hay fever represents a major cause of morbidity with impairment of quality of life for many sufferers at a time which, for most people, is the best time of the year. In the UK, symptoms which peak in June–July are largely due to grass pollen, whereas earlier symptoms peaking in April may be due to tree pollens, and in late summer/autumn due to weed pollens or moulds.[1] Perennial allergic rhinitis (frequently misdiagnosed as a 'permanent cold') results in symptoms all the year round and is due to allergy to house dust mite or domestic pets. Allergic rhinitis has been estimated to affect 15–20% of the population in westernised countries and, in common with other allergic disorders, has increased two- to three-fold over the last 20–30 years.

The diagnosis of allergic rhinitis is based on a history of typical nasal symptoms, often with associated eye symptoms, on exposure to the relevant allergens (pollens, domestic pets etc). Occupational rhinitis results from allergens encountered in the workplace, for example latex (health workers), allergens in flour (bakers), colophony (electronic solderers) and isocyanates (paint sprayers and resin manufacturers). A history suggestive of allergic rhinitis should be followed by an examination of the nose to exclude structural problems (nasal septal deflection, polyps etc), and to inspect the nasal mucosa and the character of any nasal discharge. The results of skin prick tests (measurements of allergen-specific IgE) together with the history provide helpful supportive evidence, although they may not be necessary in straightforward hay fever. Although allergy accounts for up to 60–70% of cases of perennial nasal symptoms, it is important to distinguish other conditions, including chronic rhinosinusitis, nasal polyps, other chronic inflammatory conditions (eg sarcoidosis, Wegener's granulomatosis) and rarely, mucociliary dysfunction, genetic disorders (cystic fibrosis), and benign or malignant tumours of the nose and sinuses (Table 8.1).

Table 8.1 Classification of rhinitis

Causes

Allergy (intermittent, persistent)

Infection (viral, bacterial, fungal)

Drugs (eg aspirin, beta blockers)

Hormonal (eg pregnancy, thyroid disease)

Other causes (food, irritants, emotional, acid reflux)

Idiopathic (unknown)

Differential diagnosis

Nasal polyps

Structural problems (trauma, surgery, foreign body)

Tumours (benign, malignant)

Chronic non-infectious conditions (eg sarcoidosis)

Systemic disorders (eg cystic fibrosis, mucociliary disorders)

A recent position paper, published in collaboration with the World Health Organization, has emphasised the importance of the burden of allergic rhinitis and its associated co-morbidity, especially bronchial asthma (Allergic Rhinitis and its Impact on Asthma, ARIA).[2] ARIA recommends a global classification of allergic rhinitis which is based on the duration and severity of symptoms, rather than seasonality or aetiology. It has been shown that the impaired quality of life experienced by patients with rhinitis is at least as severe or even more severe than that of patients with asthma. Since both conditions most frequently co-exist and interact, the overall impact of airway mucosal allergy may be very considerable and frequently underestimated by medical practitioners.[3]

The ARIA treatment guidelines are based on a stepwise classification (see Fig. 8.1),[2] in line with corresponding asthma guidelines (Global Initiative in Asthma: GINA, and the British Thoracic Society guidelines). The mainstay of treatment of rhinitis remains the identification and, if

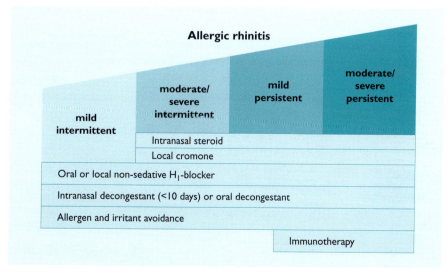

Fig 8.1   ARIA treatment guidelines for allergic rhinitis: a stepwise classification (modified from Bousquet *et al*).[2]

possible, the avoidance of provoking allergens, together with the use of H_1-antihistamines and topical nasal corticosteroids. However, a recent survey in a general practice setting in southern England found that 60% of patients continued to have bothersome symptoms despite the availability and use of these medications.[4] This suggests suboptimal treatment, through failure to recognise and avoid allergic triggers, and/or lack of explanation about the correct use of drugs, including nasal sprays. Symptom control in these patients can usually be achieved by referral to an allergist.

Immunotherapy involves the stepwise incremental injection, subcutaneously, of extracts of allergen to which the patient is sensitised.[5] Immunotherapy is highly effective in hay fever, though less so in polysensitised patients, and should not be used in chronic asthma where the risks of side effects are increased. Nonetheless, immunotherapy has been shown to confer long-term benefit[5,6] and to reduce the onset of new allergic sensitivities in children.[4] In one controlled study, it reduced the progression of rhinitis to asthma.[7] Novel approaches include the use of modified allergens and/or alternative adjuvants. The sublingual and nasal routes for immunotherapy are undoubtedly safer, although they are likely to be less effective than the conventional subcutaneous route.

Recognising the important adverse impact that rhinitis and associated sinusitis have on the quality of life, the ARIA guidelines emphasise the importance of a global approach to patients with allergic rhinitis, which may include a combination of the above strategies together with appropriate education.[2] Education should include increasing awareness and knowledge of the disease and, where appropriate, emphasis on the need for regular use of controller medication and the correct technique for the use of nasal sprays.

References

1   Van Cauwenberge P, Bachert C, Passalacqua G, Bousquet *et al.* Consensus statement on the treatment of allergic rhinitis. European Academy of Allergology and Clinical Immunology. *Allergy* 2000;**55**:116–34.

2   Allergic Rhinitis and its Impact on Asthma (ARIA). The World Health Organization Initiative, Bousquet J, van Cauwenberge P, Khaltaev NJ (eds). *J Allergy Clin Immunol* 2001;**108**:S147–334.

3   Vignolia AM, Chanez P, Bousquet J. The relationship between asthma and allergic rhinitis: exploring the basis for a common pathophysiology. *Clin Exp Allergy Rev* 2003;**3**:63–8.

4   White P, Smith H, Baker N, Davis W, Frew A. Symptom control in patients with hay fever in UK general practice: how well are we doing and is there a need for allergen immunotherapy? *Clin Exp Allergy* 1998;**28**: 266.

5   WHO position paper. Allergen immunotherapy: therapeutic vaccines for allergic diseases. Bousquet J, Lockey R, Malling HJ (eds). *Allergy* 1998;**53**(suppl 44):1–42.

6   Durham SR, Walker SM, Varga EM, Jacobson MR *et al.* Long term clinical efficacy of grass pollen immunotherapy. *New Engl J Med* 1999;**341**:468–75.

7   Moller C, Dreborg S, Ferdousi HA, Halken S *et al.* Pollen immunotherapy reduces the development of asthma in children with seasonal rhinoconjunctivitis (the PAT study). *J Allergy Clin Immunol* 2002;**109**:251–6.

Drug allergy

Drug allergy is an adverse drug reaction mediated by a specific immune response directed at the drug (or a drug breakdown product), either alone or in combination with a body protein acting as an allergen. Allergic drug reactions are either immediate or delayed, or a combination of both. Immediate drug allergy may be systemic, manifesting as hypotension with or without bronchospasm and/or angioedema, or as skin rashes that may be either local or generalised. Delayed allergic drug reactions usually affect the skin. Both anaphylaxis and severe delayed drug allergic reactions can be fatal. Allergic reactions to drugs may be classified according to Coomb's types I–IV, depending on the underlying immunological mechanism (Table 8.2). Allergic drug reactions are mediated by the immune system and are distinct from adverse drug reactions that involve toxicity, intolerance, or an abnormal response related to the principle mode of action of the drug (pharmacological side effects) (Box 8.1, overleaf). However, allergic drug responses make up a considerable proportion of adverse drug events. They may involve a genetic predisposition.[1]

Table 8.2	Mechanisms of drug allergy	
Type I	Immediate Hypersensitivity, IgE-mediated	Anaphylaxis, urticaria, angioedema, bronchospasm
Type II	Cytotoxic reactions, IgG- and IgM-mediated	Cytopenia, vasculitis
Type III	Immune complex reactions, IgG- and IgM-mediated	Serum sickness, vasculitis
Type IV	Lymphocyte-mediated reactions	Contact sensitivity Delayed onset rashes

Prevalence

As with all adverse drug reactions, the prevalence of drug allergy is hard to quantify due to under-reporting and difficulty in establishing a clear diagnosis. Spontaneous reporting of adverse drug reactions, particularly allergy/anaphylaxis, by the yellow card system, may be as low as 10% of cases. There are additional difficulties in establishing which reactions are allergic in nature. Few allergy centres in the UK are able to investigate drug allergy fully, and diagnostic tests are not straightforward. There are few extensive or rigorous published surveys of the prevalence of drug allergy. Van der Klauw and co-workers surveyed drug-induced anaphylactic reactions in the Netherlands from 1974 to 1994.[2,3] In this 20-year period, there were 40–50 cases per year of drug-induced anaphylaxis and a total of 21 anaphylactic deaths in a population of 15 million, but these are likely to be gross underestimates.

Betalactams

Penicillin and other betalactam antimicrobials are associated with either acute allergy, including acute urticaria (hives), angioedema (swelling of mucous membranes) and anaphylaxis, or delayed skin rashes which may be very severe. The acute reactions are IgE-mediated, but delayed

Box 8.1   Classification of adverse reactions to drugs

Reactions which may occur in anyone

Drug overdose
Toxic reactions linked to excess dose and/or impaired excretion or to both

Drug side effect
Undesirable pharmacological effect at recommended doses

Drug interaction
Action of a drug on the effectiveness or toxicity of another drug

Reactions which occur only in susceptible subjects

Drug intolerance
A low threshold to the normal pharmacological action of a drug

Drug idiosyncracy
A genetically determined, qualitatively abnormal reaction to a drug related to a metabolic or enzyme deficiency

Drug allergy
An immunologically mediated reaction, characterised by specificity, transferability by antibodies or lymphocytes, and recurrence on re-exposure

Pseudo-allergic reactions
A reaction with the same clinical manifestations as an allergic reaction (eg as a result of histamine release) but lacking immunological specificity

rashes are usually not. Cephalosporins and monobactams may be less often associated with allergy than the penicillins. Because patterns of antibiotic usage are rapidly changing and differ between EU countries,[4] it is important to monitor changes in specificity of betalactam allergy through pharmacosurveillance.[5]

Non-steroidal anti-inflammatory drugs

In contrast to penicillin allergy, acute allergic-type reactions to aspirin and other non-steroidal anti-inflammatory drugs (NSAIDs) are non-IgE-mediated. Their cause relates to disordered fatty acid metabolism and leukotriene production. Sensitivity to aspirin is usually associated with reactions to most, if not all, other NSAIDs. However, the novel selective cyclooxygenase inhibitors (COX2 inhibitors) are tolerated by the majority of aspirin-intolerant individuals.

Anaesthetic agents

Anaphylaxis during anaesthesia is an important area for the specialist allergist. Investigation requires expertise and should be focused in a few major allergy centres.[6] IgE-mediated reactions to drugs used to induce paralysis during anaesthesia (neuromuscular blocking drugs) represent a rare but serious cause of anaphylaxis during surgical operations. Drugs commonly implicated include suxamethonium and atracurium. The aminosteroids (eg rocuronium and vecuronium) are an increasing cause anaphylaxis. Atracurium and mivacurium also have intrinsic histamine-releasing properties that may represent an active cause of 'anaphylactoid' reactions with features identical to anaphylaxis. Suspected allergy to opiates may relate to their direct activating effects on mast cells.[6]

IgE-mediated latex allergy is another cause of reactions during anaesthesia whose prevalence in health workers and the chronically sick, eg patients with spina bifida, is increasing because of the increased use of latex gloves. Latex allergy can cause asthma, angioedema or anaphylaxis. Those who suffer from it may be at serious risk if exposed to latex during surgery or childbirth. Exposure may also occur from latex being absorbed onto the surface of starch particles used to lubricate rubber gloves.

Other drugs

Local anaesthetics are commonly suspected of causing immediate allergic reactions. Almost always such adverse events result from anxiety (eg vasovagal reactions), but they can be due to overdose, to oversensitivity to known pharmacological side effects, or a reaction to a preservative. True allergy is rare. However, it is essential to establish the diagnosis, otherwise the patient will be unable to have local anaesthetics. Skin prick tests (SPTs) to establish whether IgE sensitisation has occurred are not validated, so the gold standard test is a challenge test, which must be done in an specialist allergy centre.

Opiates, including codeine, occasionally cause allergic reactions. Angiotensin-converting enzyme (ACE) inhibitors commonly cause cough or angioedema, probably due to generation of kinins. Angioedema often involves the tongue and can be life-threatening. Anticonvulsants, antibiotics, antihypertensives and herbal remedies may cause moderate to severe delayed skin reactions which may progress to bullous eruptions, involvement of mucous membranes and even life-threatening exfoliative dermatitis. The mechanisms are unclear but are suspected of being cell-mediated and are often associated with systemic illness including liver, kidney and blood disorders. IgE tests are not relevant, although patch tests may be helpful in skilled hands.

Diagnosis

The single most important factor in making an accurate diagnosis is a detailed history (ie drugs given, duration of treatment, detailed description of reaction and its related timing). A personal or eyewitness account of events is invaluable, and every effort must be made to obtain medical records of events. For reactions under anaesthesia, the anaesthetic charts and drug charts must be obtained. True drug allergy requires prior exposure to the same or a cross-reacting drug. A detailed physical examination is necessary. The appropriate test depends on an understanding of the underlying mechanism which, unfortunately, for many drugs is unknown.

Skin prick tests

Certain drug preparations, for example penicillin major determinant (penicilloyl polylysine, PPL) and minor determinant mixture (MDM) are commercially available as skin prick solutions. Skin testing for penicillin allergy is only valuable for suspected IgE reactions and has good negative predictive value, but false-positive reactions do occur and therefore results must always be interpreted in the context of the clinical history. If not commercially available, SPTs are often performed with drugs directly from prescribed preparations, either already in solution or dissolved from tablet form (see Box 8.2, overleaf). For most drugs, the validity of such tests is unproven and both false-positive and false-negative tests occur. Skin testing for

---

Box 8.2   Immediate skin testing for diagnosing IgE-dependent allergy

Antibiotics	*Enzymes*
Penicillin	Chymopapain
Cephalosporins	Streptokinase
Anaesthetic drugs	*Chemotherapeutic drugs*
Muscle relaxants	Cisplatin
Intravenous anaesthetics	*Others*
	Insulin

False-positive and false-negative reactions may occur with these skin tests.

---

certain opiates, eg morphine and codeine, is not helpful as these drugs produce a positive skin response in all people due to a direct effect on skin mast cells not involving IgE.[7]

Patch testing

Recent evidence suggests that late-onset drug rashes may be T-cell mediated. This can be shown by patch testing. Standard patch testing (for contact dermatitis) is the province of the dermatologist. Patch testing for drugs is still in the research phase and needs to be evaluated; this is being undertaken by allergists in major centres.

Blood tests for IgE antibody

The most widely used current commercial test, the Pharmacia CAP test®, is available for a limited number of drug allergens including: amoxicilloyl, ampicilloyl, penicilloyl G, penicilloyl V, cefaclor, and suxamethonium. These tests may be unreliable and should be carefully interpreted in the light of the history. Their availability is confined to regional laboratories.

Drug provocation tests

Direct challenge with specific drugs should be undertaken at specialist allergy centres only when investigations have been exhausted and the diagnosis remains in doubt. The challenge should be designed either to implicate or exclude a drug, or to identify a suitable alternative agent (eg cephalosporin in a penicillin-sensitive patient). The risk/benefit must be assessed in every case; in the case of anaphylaxis, challenge should be avoided unless no suitable alternative exists. These tests should only be carried out in a specialist centre by staff trained in the treatment of anaphylaxis.

Other tests

In an acute severe reaction, blood should be drawn at 1–2 hours after onset to test for circulating tryptase (a protein that is secreted by activated mast cells) levels. A raised serum tryptase at 1–2 hours confirms that either IgE- or non-IgE-mediated mast cell degranulation has occurred. Basophil activation tests for immediate sensitivity and T lymphocyte activation (delayed reactions) are at present not generally available and are confined to research use.[8,9]

Treatment

In allergic reactions to drugs, the immediate need is for emergency treatment of the reaction, especially in the case of anaphylaxis. It is essential to withdraw the offending drug immediately, which means identifiying it, but this may be difficult when patients are taking several drugs. It is also important to identify a safe alternative for the patient. Ideally, the identity of the offending drug should be confirmed afterwards, but this is not always possible.

Current concerns: test availability and validity

Skin testing for penicillin, neuromuscular blocking drugs and anaesthetic agents is well validated, but many drug allergy diagnostic tests are not. Tests must be of proven validity, ie the incidence of false-positive and false-negative results must be within acceptable limits, and these data are not available for many drugs. There is no suitable reference test or guidelines covering availability, validity and protocols for drug allergy tests, so drug challenge tests remain the gold standard. Patients should be referred to specialist allergy centres, where experience is concentrated and evidence-based guidelines can be developed.

References

1 Vervloet D, Durham SR. Adverse reactions to drugs. In: Durham SR (ed) *ABC of allergies*. London: BMJ Books, 1998:48–51.

2 van der Klauw MM, Wilson JH, Stricker BH. Drug-associated anaphylaxis: 20 years of reporting in The Netherlands (1974–1994) and review of the literature. *Clin Exp Allergy* 1996;**26**:1355–63.

3 van der Klauw MM, Wilson JH, Stricker BH. Drug-associated agranulocytosis: 20 years of reporting in The Netherlands (1974-1994). *Am J Hematol* 1998;**57**:206–11.

4 Cars O, Molstad S, Melander A. Variation in antibiotic use in the European Union. *Lancet* 2001;**357**:1851–3.

5 Blanca, M. Allergic reactions to penicillins. A changing world? *Allergy* 1995;**50**:777–82.

6 The Association of Anaesthetists of Great Britain and Northern Ireland and the British Society for Allergy and Clinical Immunology. *Suspected anaphylactic reaction associated with anaesthesia*, 3rd edn. London: Association of Anaesthetists, BSACI, 2003.

7 Nasser SM, Ewan PW. Opiate-sensitivity: clinical characteristics and the role of skin prick testing. *Clin Exp Allergy* 2001;**31**:1014–20.

8 Crockard AD, Ennis M. Laboratory-based allergy diagnosis: should we go with the flow? *Clin Exp Allergy* 2001;**31**:975–7.

9 Pichler WJ, Schnyder B, Zanni M, Hari Y, von Greyers S. Role of T cells in drug allergies. *Allergy* 1998;**53**:225–32.

Food allergy and intolerance

Food allergy is the cause of much controversy. IgE-mediated reactions are fairly well defined and straightforward for the allergist, although there is much to learn in relation to newly emerged disorders, but these problems are difficult for GPs and non-specialists. However, reactions due to other mechanisms (often referred to as 'food intolerance') are much more difficult because of lack of consensus on definition and the lack of reliable and easily applied tests.

Food reactions that relate to enzyme deficiency will not be discussed here. Enzyme deficiency apart, food reactions may be toxic or non-toxic. Toxic reactions do not relate to allergy but occur in anyone who ingests a sufficient quantity of a specific type of food. Toxic 'pharmacological' reactions to foods are well known; for example symptom responses to caffeine and alcohol. True toxic reactions are more complex and the cause may be difficult to trace. For example, it took some time to link an outbreak of a life-threatening multi-system illness in Spain in 1982 to the ingestion of illegally produced and contaminated cooking oil. Reactions indistinguishable from IgE-mediated food allergy can sometimes occur when histamine is released directly from foods. For example, scombroid food poisoning is due to prior bacterial spoilage of fish (eg tuna) which causes release of sufficiently high levels of histamine to induce symptoms. Conversely, non-toxic food reactions are specific to the sufferer. The best understood food reactions are those that occur immediately (within one hour) of food ingestion. Immunological responses (IgE-mediated type 1 hypersensitivity reactions) underlie the majority of such reactions. Delayed reactions are poorly understood and for the majority the mechanism is unknown.

Immediate reactions to foods (IgE-mediated or classical food allergy)

Immediate reactions to food are due to the interaction of food allergen with specific IgE bound to mast cells (see Chapter 1).

Prevalence

Lack of definition of mechanisms and lack of expertise in diagnosis makes it difficult to define the overall prevalence of food allergy. However, it is clear that the prevalence is high, and rising rapidly in the developed world. Data suggesting that 1.8–3.2% of the population have food reactions must underestimate the position now, as peanut and milk allergy alone account for more than this.[1,2] Peanut allergy was previously rare, with only a few case reports, but allergy to both peanuts and tree nuts has risen substantially in the last decade, with the first report of a major series in 1993–4.[3] Tariq *et al* examined all children born on the Isle of Wight in a single year, 1989. By the age of four, 0.5% (one in 200) had suffered an allergic reaction to peanut.[4] Four years later, 1.6% (one in 70) were allergic and 3.2% sensitised, ie a trebling of peanut allergy in this period.[5] The Avon Longitudinal Study of Parents and Children (ALSPAC) produced similar findings.[6] In the USA, where peanut consumption is higher, 7.2% of children and adults are sensitised.[7] Clinical practice shows that allergy to fruits and vegetables, also previously rare, has increased rapidly over the last five years but there are no data on prevalence.

Which foods cause allergy?

Almost any food can cause allergy. However, a few foods cause most reactions, particularly egg, milk and peanuts, but also tree nuts, fish, shellfish, soya and wheat.[8] Fruits and vegetables now need to be added to this list.

Clinical features

The clinical features vary from mild reactions through to severe, including anaphylaxis. Mild reactions typically include facial erythema, urticaria and angioedema, but may also include generalised cutaneous features. Respiratory symptoms are important in food allergy. A moderate reaction includes slight laryngeal oedema (a sensation of closing up of the throat) or mild asthma. Vomiting may occur, especially in children. In severe reactions, respiratory features dominate, with acute severe dyspnoea usually due to laryngeal oedema but also to asthma. This may progress rapidly to asphyxia and respiratory arrest, with hypotension secondary to the respiratory problem.[3] Onset is soon after ingestion of the food, usually within 10 minutes, and mostly within 30 minutes. Severe reactions begin early and progress rapidly. Early recognition and treatment is mandatory.

Peanut and tree nut allergy

Allergy to peanuts develops in young children[4] who almost always (96%) have a history of atopy (most commonly eczema, followed by asthma, allergic rhinitis, egg and milk allergy).[3,9] The median age of onset of peanut allergy is two years. Tree nut allergy develops later in childhood. There is usually a family history of allergy (maternal more often than paternal), and an increased prevalence of peanut allergy in siblings of 7%.[10]

Although this is a major cause of severe and fatal reactions, the clinical spectrum varies greatly.[9] The majority of patients' worst ever reactions to peanuts and nuts are mild (51%) and involve mainly cutaneous features.[3,9] However, 35–40% of patients' worst ever reactions involve asthma and/or laryngeal oedema, and 7–12% have life-threatening dyspnoea and/or hypotension.[9,11]

Severe and fatal reactions to food

Food allergy is a major cause of fatal reactions[12] and the most common cause of childhood anaphylaxis in the UK,[13] and peanut allergy is the most common cause of fatal and near-fatal reactions to foods at all ages.[14] Fatalities and severe reactions to nuts are most common amongst adolescents and adults,[15] but a recent US survey found that one-third of fatalities (94% due to peanuts and tree nuts) occurred in children.[14]

A recent UK population study of children from 1990 to 2000 found that only eight died because of an allergic reaction to a food.[16] Some experts believe that this study seriously underestimated the risk because some deaths may have been wrongly attributed to asthma alone;[17,18] comparison with other data also shows the figure for severe food reactions in this study to be an underestimate.[18,19]

In a series of patients who suffered fatal or near-fatal reactions to food, those who died received adrenaline late, and patients who survived mostly received adrenaline within 30 minutes of allergen ingestion.[15] The implication is that patients should carry emergency medication which is available for early self-administration, and that they should be trained in its indications and use.

Anaphylactic deaths due to food allergy usually occur in patients who know they have a food allergy, but have been unable to obtain medical advice either because of GPs' lack knowledge of allergy, or because there was no allergy service available locally.

Management of nut allergy

The diagnosis of peanut allergy creates alarm in parents and GPs because of the risk of fatal reactions. Having gone through a phase of under-management, there is now a tendency for GPs to prescribe an adrenaline auto-injector for all patients. This is inappropriate, as there is a spectrum of severity. It is difficult for non-specialists to manage these patients, and they should be seen in major allergy centres.

Patients who are aware of the diagnosis and avoid nuts still have a 50% incidence of further reactions.[20] A management plan has now been developed and evaluated in 567 patients.[9] This involved providing detailed written and verbal advice on avoidance, emergency medication based on assessment of severity of reaction, training and re-training in its use, and training of school staff.[21] This was effective: 15% of patients had further reactions, but most were trivial or mild, and only three were severe enough to require self-administered adrenaline, which was always effective. Other allergies were also controlled, with particular attention given to asthma control. Management must be integrated and comprehensive, and must consist of more than prescribing adrenaline.[22,23]

This approach to management is applicable to most types of food allergy. The reactions that cause the greatest risk in severe and fatal cases are acute laryngeal oedema and asthma.

Oral allergy syndrome

Oral allergy syndrome occurs in some hay fever sufferers and is characterised by immediate itching and swelling of the mouth and throat after the ingestion of certain fruits, nuts and vegetables. It occurs because of the presence of IgE antibodies directed towards common cross-reacting proteins (eg profilins) that exist both in the pollens and the foods concerned. Thus, people sensitive to silver birch pollen can react to raw (but not cooked) apple, peach, cherry, hazel nut, carrot and other foods; those with mugwort (weed) pollen hay fever may react to raw celery and carrots. This disorder used to be rare but has become common in the last five years. Previously it was mild, but now some patients have more severe respiratory difficulty.

Food allergy in latex allergy

An association between food and non-food allergens is also seen in latex allergy.[24] Allergy to natural rubber latex can cause urticaria, conjunctivitis, rhinitis, asthma and anaphylaxis. Individuals allergic to latex may develop allergy to banana, kiwi, avocado, mango and chestnuts, due to cross-reacting allergens in these foods.

Egg and milk allergy

Egg and milk allergy are common in children. In the majority, reactions are mild to moderate, but a small proportion have anaphylaxis. There is a strong association with other atopic diseases, particularly eczema, asthma and rhinitis. Egg and milk allergy resolve in almost 90% of children, usually by the age of five.

Diagnosis

Tests for specific IgE antibodies to foods are useful but must be interpreted in the light of the history. When compared with results of double-blind placebo-controlled food challenge, the positive predictive accuracy of skin prick tests (SPTs) is less than 50% (false-positives are common) although negative predictive accuracy is better at 95% (false-negatives are rare). This is because sensitisation (the presence of food-specific IgE antibody) can occur without clinical allergy.[25] This means that negative SPT results are more useful in excluding IgE-mediated food allergies than positive SPT results are in diagnosing it. Positive skin test responses therefore need to be viewed in conjunction with the clinical history to ensure that inappropriate food exclusion is not enforced.

Studies have compared the degree of positivity of both the SPT and the measurement of serum specific IgE (radioallergosorbent test (RAST)) with food challenge. This has allowed the definition of cut-off thresholds in an attempt to improve the positive predictive value of the test.[26]

Hospital-based supervised food challenge may be required in patients of any age when there is neither unequivocal recent reaction history nor above-threshold positive test. Children may outgrow food allergy and may need to be tested in hospital before reintroducing the food into their diet.

The dietitian's role in immediate food allergy

It is not easy simply to avoid foods. Patients need to be taught how to interpret the list of ingredients on the labels of manufactured foods. For example, they may not know that the terms 'whey' and 'casein' indicate the presence of milk. Also, food labelling is not completely comprehensive: confectionary often has no list of ingredients and many foods, such as bakery products and sandwiches, may be completely unlabelled. To add to the confusion, possible contamination at sites of manufacture means that many manufactured foods have 'may contain' (eg nuts) labels on them. For patients with food allergy, eating away from home can also be a major problem.

An appropriately trained dietitian is an important member of any allergy clinic team. S/he can help the patient avoid the problem foods as completely as possible, finding alternatives to avoided foods (eg milk or wheat) where necessary. An important parallel role is to ensure that those with established food allergy, especially growing children, have a nutritionally adequate diet. The provision of recipes, advice when eating out, and general encouragement are additional measures that are helpful. In certain situations, s/he may need to arrange for food challenge tests. An allergy department should have the services of both adult and paediatric dietitians.

Delayed reactions to foods (food intolerance)

Food intolerance is a more difficult and poorly defined area, where there is much less evidence on which to base practice. Because the underlying mechanisms are largely undefined, there are no established tests, and diagnosis is made mainly on the basis of food exclusion and reintroduction.[27] Symptoms vary and may include gastrointestinal symptoms such as bloating and flatulence.

Reactions to cow's milk in children

Late onset non-IgE-mediated reactions to cow's milk are not uncommon.[28] A study of children tested by cow's milk exclusion and challenge showed three distinct patterns of response.[29] In one third, there were responses typical of immediate food allergy (vomiting, diarrhoea, urticaria/angioedema, rhinitis or asthma) occurring within an hour, and associated with high levels of IgE antibodies to milk. Half of the total fell into an intermediate group that required a larger milk dose to induce symptoms (vomiting, diarrhoea, colic and an association with failure to thrive) that commenced between two and 24 hours after challenge. The remainder (20%) took between one and five days to react and generally required repeated ingestion of milk to induce symptoms.

Coeliac disease

Coeliac disease is an immunological disorder caused by gluten sensitivity, which is not IgE-mediated. It is managed by gastroenterologists and is not the province of the allergist (except to recognise and refer on).

Characteristic features are :

- typical symptoms
- chronic lymphocytic inflammation and villous atrophy on intestinal biopsy
- clinical remission and resolution of the biopsy changes following introduction of a gluten-free diet.

Atopic eczema

According to evidence from double-blind placebo-controlled food challenges (DBPCFCs), 40% of infants and young children with moderate to severe eczema have evidence of food allergy. Whilst there is much evidence for the role of food-specific IgE in the pathogenesis of eczema, there is poor correlation between these results and the DBPCFC. Other children with eczema with DBPCFC evidence of intolerance to specific food proteins show no evidence of IgE sensitisation to that protein, suggesting that other mechanisms are operative.[30] Immediate symptom responses on DBPCFC tend to equate with positive SPT (IgE), whilst delayed symptom responses tend to equate to a positive patch test (T-cell response). This suggests that a variety of immune responses are operating in atopic eczema.

Urticaria

The vasoactive amine content of foods, especially the histamine and histamine-releasing content, has been linked to urticaria in a subset of patients. Food dyes and food additives only occasionally cause urticaria.

Irritable bowel syndrome

Exclusion of a range of foodstuffs has been claimed to relieve the symptoms of a subgroup of patients with irritable bowel syndrome (IBS). In one study, symptom improvement was reported in half of the patients, and open food challenge identified one or more symptom-provoking foods.[31] In other studies, beneficial response rates ranging from 15 to 67% of subjects to food exclusion have been reported, with randomised placebo-controlled food challenges identifying specific food precipitants (the most common being milk, wheat and eggs) in 6–58% of subjects. Overall, these studies suggest that a subgroup of IBS patients may respond to therapeutic dietary manipulation, but this is usually an adjunct to other treatment. Further studies are needed. In patients suspected to have irritable bowel syndrome, other physical disorders should be excluded, usually by a gastroenterologist.

Crohn's disease

Inflammatory bowel disease must remain the province of the gastroenterologist. Some patients with Crohn's disease have been shown to improve on specially selected diets, the condition then being exacerbated by specific food reintroduction.

Hyperactivity

Although many studies have attempted to show a relationship between attention deficit hyperactivity disorder (ADHD) and food additives and/or salicylates, convincing proof of this relationship remains to be established. This is an area for further research.

Migraine and epilepsy

The relationship of foods to central nervous system disorders has been the subject of much controversy. A study of the effect of food exclusions was carried out in children with co-existing migraine and epilepsy, or epilepsy alone.[32] Many in the first group responded with a reduction in migraine or epilepsy. During a placebo-controlled challenge phase, various symptoms, including epilepsy, were provoked by several foods. It was noted that children with epilepsy but not migraine did not respond to the food exclusion regimes. Further studies are needed.

Multiple symptoms

Some patients present with multiple non-specific symptoms, which may include arthralgia, fatigue, headaches, bowel upset and difficulty in concentration. Such presentations are often given the label of food intolerance, but there is little evidence to support this at present, apart from anecdotal claims of improvement in a few patients where certain foods have been excluded. The validation of such presentations as food-related is difficult because of lack of understanding of the mechanisms and presentations of food intolerance. Some patients have psychological problems; in others, a secondary problem arises with weight loss following inappropriate dietary exclusion. A sympathetic approach is required. A specialist allergist has an important role in offering these patients the advice they seek, as often they have been unable to obtain it elsewhere. It is essential that the allergist excludes other physical disorders which may be mislabelled as food intolerance.

The dietitian's role in food intolerance

A trained dietitian is in a strong position to provide help, advice and encouragement with the inevitable nutritional and social compromises that result from the need to follow an exclusion diet. In the case of non-IgE-mediated food problems, the dietitian is also likely to be involved in the diagnostic process. Until standardised tests or diagnostic methods have been established, this will remain a difficult area. Particularly taxing are patients or parents who present with the preconception that food intolerance (not infrequently self-diagnosed and reinforced by reading literature or consulting alternative practitioners) underlies a particular set of symptoms. Such preconceptions about symptom causation may often remain unconfirmed in spite of careful and sympathetic attempts to reproduce the circumstances of their occurrence.

References

1 Young E, Stoneham MD, Petruckevitch A, Barton J, Rona R. A population study of food intolerance. *Lancet* 1994;**343**(8906):1127–30.

2 Kanny G, Moneret-Vautrin DA, Flabbee J, Beaudouin E *et al.* Population study of food allergy in France. *J Allergy Clin Immunol* 2001;**108**(1):133–40.

3 Ewan PW. Clinical study of peanut and nut allergy in 62 consecutive patients: new features and associations. *BMJ* 1996;**312**:1074–8.

4 Tariq SM, Stevens M, Matthews W, Ridout S *et al.* Cohort study of peanut and tree nut sensitisation by age of 4 years. *BMJ* 1996;**313**:514–7.

5 Grundy J, Matthews S, Bateman B, Dean T, Arshad SH. Rising prevalence of allergy to peanut in children: data from 2 sequential cohorts. *J Allergy Clin Immunol* 2002;**110**:784–9.

6 ALSPAC website: www.AlspacExt/pressrelease/peanut%20allergy.htm

7 Chiu L, Sampson HA, Sicherer SH. Estimation of the sensitisation rate to peanut by prick skin test in the general population: results from the National Health and Nutrition Examination Survey 1988-94. *J Allergy Clin Immunol* 2001;**107**:5192.

8 Bock SA, Sampson HA Atkins FM, Zeiger RS *et al.* Double blind, placebo-controlled food challenge (DBPCFC) as an office procedure: a manual. *J Allergy Clin Imunol* 1988;**82**:986–97.

9 Ewan PW, Clark AT. Long-term prospective observational study of the outcome of a management plan in patients with peanut and nut allergy referred to a regional allergy centre. *Lancet* 2001;**357**:111.

10 Hourihane JO, Dean TP, Warner JO. Peanut allergy in relation to heredity, maternal diet, and other atopic diseases: results of a questionnaire survey, skin prick testing and food challenges. *BMJ* 1996;**313**:518–21.

11 Clark AT. Development of peanut and nut allergy; clinical and immunological findings. MD thesis, University of London, 2003.

12 Pumphrey RS. Lessons for management of anaphylaxis from a study of fatal reactions. *Clin Exp Allergy* 2000;**30**:1144–50.

13 Alves B, Sheikh A. Age specific aetiology of anaphylaxis. *Arch Dis Child* 2001;**85**:348.

14 Bock SA, Munoz-Furlong A, Sampson HA. Fatalities due to anaphylactic reactions to foods. *J Allergy Clin Immunol* 2001;**107**:191–3.

15 Sampson HA, Mendelson L, Rosen JP. Fatal and near-fatal anaphylactic reactions to food in children and adolescents. *N Engl J Med* 1992;**327**:380–4.

16 MacDougall CF, Cant AJ, Colver AF. How dangerous is food allergy in childhood? The incidence of severe and fatal allergic reactions across the UK and Ireland. *Arch Dis Child* 2002;**86**:236–9.

17 Hourihane JO, Reading D, Smith P, Lack G *et al.* Incidence of severe and fatal reactions to foods. *Arch Dis Child* 2002;**87**:450–1.

18 Clark AT, Ewan PW. Food allergy in childhood. Have the dangers been underestimated? *Arch Dis Child* 2003;**88**:79–81.

19 Sheikh A, Alves B. Hospital admissions for acute anaphylaxis: time trend study. *BMJ* 2000;**320**:1441.

20 Hourihane JO, Kilburn SA, Dean P, Warner JO. Clinical characterisitcs of peanut allergy. *Clin Exp Allergy* 1997;**27**:634–9.

21 Vickers DW, Maynard L, Ewan PW. Management of children with potential anaphylactic reactions in the community: a training package and proposals for good practice. *Clin Exp Allergy* 1997;**27**:898–903.

22 Hourihane JO. Community management of severe allergies must be integrated and comprehensive, and must consist of more than just epinephrine. *Allergy* 2001;**56**:1023–5.

23 Hourihane JO. Recent advances in peanut allergy. *Curr Opin Allergy Clin Immunol* 2002;**2**:227–31.

24 Blanco C. Latex–fruit syndrome. *Curr Allergy Asthma Rep* 2003;**3**:47–53.

25 Clark AT, Ewan PW. Interpretation of tests for nut allergy in a thousand patients in relation to allergy or tolerance. *Clin Exp Allergy* 2003;**33** (in press).

26 Roberts G, Lack G. Food allergy: Getting more out of your skin prick tests. *Clin Exp Allergy* 2000;**30**: 1495–8.

27 Brostoff J, Challacombe SJ (eds). *Food allergy and intolerance*, 2nd edn. London: Saunders, 2002.

28 Sampson HA, Anderson JA. Summary and recommendations. Classification of gastrointestinal manifestations due to immunologic reactions to foods in infants and young children. *J Pediatr Gastroenterol* 2000;**30**:S87–S94.

29 Hill DJ, Firer MA *et al.* Manifestations of milk allergy in infancy: clinical and immunological findings. *J Pediatr* 1986;**109**: 270–6.

30 Majamaa H, Moisio P, Holm K *et al.* Cow's milk allergy: diagnostic accuracy of skin prick and patch tests and specific IgE. *Allergy* 1999;**54**:346–51.

31 Nanda R, James R, Smith H, Dudley CR, Jewell DP. Food intolerance and the irritable bowel syndrome. *Gut* 1989;**30**:1099–104.

32 Egger J, Carter CM, Soothill JF, Wilson J. Oligoantigenic diet treatment of children with epilepsy and migraine. *J Pediatr* 1989;**114**:51–8.

Allergy and the skin

A wide range of skin diseases can produce itching and redness associated with swelling, features which are often presumed to reflect the presence of an allergic reaction. The allergist has a role to play in urticaria, angioedema and atopic dermatitis, mainly by determining allergic and other triggers. The role of allergic triggers can be very variable and is important to determine precisely. It can be difficult to determine in atopic dematitis. Many drug reactions have cutaneous manifestations which can mimic a variety of diseases with known allergic or non-allergic aetiologies. Also, some drugs/chemicals can have direct, non-immunological effects on skin, inducing degranulation of mast cells resulting in erythema, urticaria and/or angioedema. Urticaria and angioedema can thus be IgE- or non-IgE-mediated, and the allergist has a role to play in both. In atopic dermatitis the role is to determine allergic triggers. Other forms of eczema are dealt with by dermatologists.

Urticaria

Urticaria ('hives', nettle rash) and angioedema (swelling of the deeper subcutaneous tissue) are common disorders. Urticarial processes can be subdivided into three types:

1 *Allergic:* urticarial weals develop on exposure to allergens (eg foods, drugs, animal danders, pollens or latex rubber).

2 *Physical:* external stimuli such as change in temperature, pressure on the skin, shearing (scratching) force, or sunlight-induced mast cell degranulation cause weal and flare formation. Cholinergic urticaria can develop after such stimuli as a rise in body temperature, emotional stress or exercise.

3 *Idiopathic:* the process mimics allergic urticaria but no allergic basis can be determined.

Chronic idiopathic urticaria accounts for the vast majority of reactions. In some cases, auto (self-directed) antibodies are generated that are directed to IgE or IgE receptors on mast cells to activate them, in a similar way to that observed in classical allergic responses. In autoimmune and other forms of idiopathic urticaria, the weals are longer lasting and show a variable response to antihistamine therapy.

Angioedema

Angioedema may occur alone, with urticaria, or with a variety of other symptoms as part of a multi-system disorder (ranging from hay fever, to food or drug allergy, to anaphylaxis). The potential causes of each type vary.

Angioedema can be often severe, causing asphyxia if it involves the tongue or the larynx, or it may be a manifestation of anaphylaxis. An allergist is best placed to manage such patients, whether the disease is IgE-mediated, as in food allergy, or due to other mechanisms, as with drugs such as ACE inhibitors. Glottal oedema is often isolated and causes severe dyspnoea or difficulty speaking. The most common causes are drug-induced or idiopathic. Laryngeal oedema is common in food allergy but occurs in other allergies, and is one of the features of anaphylaxis.

It is important to determine whether there are specific triggers or whether urticaria and angio-edema are idiopathic. An allergist can therefore act as a resource for GPs or dermatologists in these disorders. Isolated urticaria is often dealt with primarily by dermatologists, but allergists will have a role in some patients, eg if there is associated angioedema or if an allergic cause is a possibility.

First-line treatment for angioedema and urticaria is with oral antihistamines, but sometimes high doses or a combination of non-sedative drugs by day and sedative antihistamines at night are required. Other drugs, including oral steroids or occasionally immunosuppressives, may be needed.

Glottal oedema

Treatment for glottal oedema is described in Chapter 10, p 79.

Hereditary angioedema

In hereditary angioedema (HAE), attacks of angioedema occur at three sights: cutaneous; intestinal, presenting with abdominal pain due to sub-acute intestinal obstruction; and laryngeal, which can be fatal. This disorder is due to deficiency of the complement component C1 esterase inhibitor, resulting in uncontrolled complement activation and generation of mediators causing capillary leak. Intermittent attacks occur. There is a typical presentation, and this diagnosis should also be suspected from the history.

Confirmatory tests include measurement of C1 esterase inhibitor (by antigenetic ± functional assay), and C4.

Management requires experience and this rare disorder should ideally be managed in major allergy centres treating reasonable numbers of patients. Treatment includes prophylactic therapy with danazol or, in patients unsuitable for this, an infusion of fresh frozen plasma or of purified C1 inhibitor can be used to stop acute severe attacks.

Atopic dermatitis (atopic eczema)

Atopic dermatitis (or atopic eczema) is a chronic recurrent inflammation of the skin characterised by intense itching with erythema, dryness and/or weeping. It affects different body sites at different ages. In a small baby it may involve the whole body. In a crawling child, it may affect extensor surfaces. In toddlers, children and adults, it has a predilection for the flexures. Affected individuals often have other atopic disorders such as allergic rhinitis, asthma or food allergy, and commonly several disorders are present in the same patient. Different types of allergic reaction can be elicited with different types of skin challenge. Prick test evokes an IgE-mediated degranulation of mast cells resulting in weal and flare; patch testing on slightly abraded or tape-striped skin evokes both immediate and delayed eczematous reactions. A number of factors can exacerbate or provoke atopic eczema. These include allergy to dietary substances (especially in young children), or airborne allergens including house dust mites, animal furs and pollens. The causal role of dust mites has been clearly demonstrated in controlled trials of allergen avoidance. The role of food allergy is often hard to determine in individual cases but some individuals show great benefit from avoidance of selected foods such as milk and/or eggs. Other aggravating/provoking factors include skin surface microbes (eg staphylococci). In many patients, eczema is aggravated by emotional upheaval, changes in humidity and temperature, as well as contact with synthetic fibres (nylon) or wool.

Atopic eczema may be an isolated problem but more often is part of multi-system allergic disease, with co-existent asthma, allergic rhinitis and food allergy, and the particular contribution of the allergist is to provide a global approach, identify allergic triggers and give advice on avoidance. This is an important aspect of management, which is usually not otherwise provided.

Diagnosis

Investigations such as skin prick tests or measurement of serum specific IgE can provide supporting evidence for a particular allergic cause for a skin complaint. However, recourse to a detailed history is essential, because IgE sensitisation can occur without symptoms. Interpretation of positive tests is important. Thus, requesting tests for IgE in the serum eg by RAST, is inappropriate unless results are interpreted by a doctor with allergy training and in conjunction with the history. Many patients who eventually reach an allergy clinic have had large number of RASTs but the results have been misinterpreted. Avoidance of possible causes is a way of establishing an underlying allergic response.

Contact dermatitis

Contact dermatitis may be due to allergy, irritation or both. This disorder is usually managed by a dermatologist, but allergists need to recognise it. Contact dermatitis on body sites other than the hands is usually due to allergic mechanisms. However, on the hands the distinction between allergic and irritant contact dermatitis can be difficult to make but is very important.

Irritant contact dermatitis of the hands is one of the most common occupational skin diseases. The hand skin of almost all people can be irritated by exposure to sufficiently aggressive solvents/surfactants. Chronic irritation produces an eczematous dermatitis, which can be indistinguishable from an allergic contact dermatitis. In general, the pattern and distribution of the eczematous dermatitis suggests an exogenous and possible allergic cause. The pattern and distribution of the skin reaction is likely to match the sites of contact with external agents such as items of clothing, cosmetics, watches and jewellery, medicaments etc. Common sensitising agents include nickel, perfumes/fragrances, ingredients in rubber (gloves and shoes), dye substances and formaldehyde releasing agents. The standard method for testing is the patch test (provided by dermatologists) which evokes a 48-hour eczematous reaction. The patch test shows the presence of sensitised T lymphocytes. Contact dermatitis is not due to IgE antibody. Certain substances are converted to sensitising allergen through the action of ultraviolet light (photocontact sensitisers).

Venom allergy (allergy to stings)

Hymenoptera (bee or wasp (vespid)) stings may cause allergic reactions. The incidence of stings in most studies is less than 0.2%, and only a minority of these cause allergic reactions. In the UK, bee sting allergy (honeybee) occurs mainly in beekeepers, their relatives or neighbours, ie in those exposed and frequently stung. In contrast, wasp venom allergy, which is much more common than bee venom allergy in the UK, occurs with random occasional stings (Fig 8.2). This disorder is important because of the risk of fatal and near-fatal anaphylaxis, and because venom immunotherapy is highly effective. The disorder requires advice from a specialist allergist.

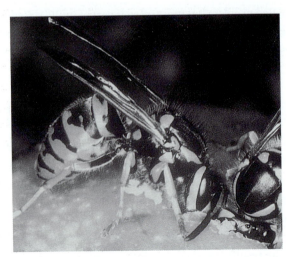

Fig 8.2 The wasp is the most common insect to cause anaphylaxis in the UK. (Reproduced from *BMJ* 1998;**316**:1365–8, with permission from the BMJ Publishing Group.)

Clinical features

Reactions may be local or systemic.

Large local reactions (LLR)   These are local swellings at the site of the sting, without systemic allergic features. It is important to clarify from the history that these are indeed large, eg involving the whole forearm. These are not usually a precursor of systemic reactions.

Systemic reactions (SR)   These vary widely in severity from systemic cutaneous reactions to anaphylaxis.[1] Systemic cutaneous reactions consist of erythema, pruritus and generalised urticaria with or without angioedema. In anaphylaxis, reactions are of rapid onset (typically, a few up to 15 minutes from the sting) and of variable presentation. Most commonly, the initial features are cutaneous followed by features of hypotension, with light-headedness, fainting or collapse. Some patients develop respiratory symptoms due to either asthma or laryngeal oedema, but this is less frequent than in food-induced allergic reactions. However, a few patients have little or no warning, eg slight cutaneous features, and then rapidly collapse and lose consciousness. In severe reactions, patients often feel that they are going to die (a sense of impending doom). Less common features are conjunctivitis, rhinitis and gastrointestinal reactions (vomiting, abdominal pain). Rarely, patients have retrosternal chest pain, incontinence or fitting (restricted to some of those with profound hypotension). It is helpful in assessing patients to classify systemic reactions as mild, moderate or severe.

Diagnosis

This is based on the history confirmed by allergen skin-testing (either prick or intradermal) and measurement of venom-specific IgE antibody in serum. Pitfalls are incorrect identification of the insect by the patient, a high incidence of double positive venom IgE (bee and wasp) yet clinical allergy to only one insect[2] and negative IgE to venom. It should be remembered that 20–25% of adults who have no reaction to a sting have a positive test for specific IgE. The serum venom IgE is negative in up to 20% of skin-test positive subjects, and neither test alone will detect all patients; it is therefore important to do both. Some patients with negative IgE to venoms have been shown to have venom IgE by immunoblotting techniques.

Natural history

It is essential to understand this in order to decide on appropriate management. The placebo wing of the first double-blind study of pure venom immunotherapy revealed that 40% of untreated patients with systemic reactions do not react to subsequent stings.[3] This has been borne out by subsequent studies of response to field or challenge stings. The incidence of further reactions varies widely but can be as low as 20%, with an overall mean reaction rate of 45%. Children with cutaneous systemic reactions are at even lower risk (about 10%) of further systemic reactions, and only a 0.4% incidence of more severe reactions.[4] The prognosis is best for those with the milder systemic reactions, for children, for those with wasp allergy, and when the interval between stings is longer.[5] Patients are commonly told 'your next reaction will be worse', but this is not true.

Acute management

The key drug for anaphylactic reactions is intramuscular adrenaline (epinephrine) which should be given early.

Further management

The risk of a further reaction will depend on:

(i)   the previous history

(ii)   the natural history of the disease

(iii)   the immunological status of the patient

(iv)   the risk of a further sting

(v)   the interval from the last sting.

Patients may be given medication to carry for self-treatment or venom immunotherapy. Medication may include an adrenaline auto-injector (Epipen®), if they are considered at risk of a severe reaction, or oral quick-acting antihistamines. It is essential that those prescribing Epipen® also train patients in its use. Ideally, a written treatment plan should be given to patients, outlining reactions of different severities and their treatment (to prevent inappropriate use of Epipen®).

Venom immunotherapy

Venom immunotherapy (VIT) is highly effective, protecting about 95% of patients with vespid venom allergy and 80–90% of those allergic to bee venom.[3,6] Quality of life is also improved.[7] The main disadvantage of immunotherapy is the risk of side effects (which are more likely with bee than wasp VIT), but the cost and time commitment should also be considered. Conventional VIT is given with an initial course of incremental injections of pure venom, then maintenance therapy at monthly to three-monthly intervals, usually for three years in the UK. This is best done in a specialist allergy centre where many patients are being treated, with good systems for monitoring and early treatment of systemic reactions. Venom immunotherapy should not be done as a 'one-off' or by doctors not experienced in IT. The appropriate venom must be used (see pitfalls in Diagnosis above). Guidelines in the UK suggest that immunotherapy as a preventive treatment should be reserved for severe and some moderate systemic reactions.[8]

VIT results in a shift from the Th-2 dominant to a Th-1 dominant cytokine profile,[9] and early induction of the protective cytokine interleukin (IL)-10 seems important in inducing specific immune tolerance.[10,11]

References

1   Ewan PW. Venom allergy. *BMJ* 1998;**316**:1365–8.

2   Egner W, Ward C, Brown DL, Ewan PW. The incidence and clinical significance of specific IgE to both wasp (Vespula) and bee (Apis) venom in the same patient. *Clin Exp Allergy*, 1998;**28**:26–34.

3   Hunt KJ, Valentine MD, Sobotka AK, Benton AW *et al*. A controlled trial of immunotherapy in insect hypersensitivity. *N Engl J Med* 1978;**299**:157–61.

4   Valentine MD, Schuberth KC, Kagey-Sobotka A, Graft DF *et al.* The value of immunotherapy with venom in children with allergy to insect stings. *N Engl J Med* 1990;**323**:1601–3.

5   Golden DBK, Marsh DG, Freidhoff LR, Kwiterovich KA *et al.* Natural history of Hymenoptera venom sensitivity in adults. *J Allergy Clin Immunol* 1997;**100**:760–6.

6   Muller U, Mosbech H. Position paper: immunotherapy with Hymenoptera venoms. *Allergy* 1993;**48**:37–46.

7   Oude Elberink JNG, de Monchy JGR, Golden DBK, Brouwer JP *et al.* Development and validation of a health-related quality-of-life questionnaire in patients with yellow jacket allergy. *J Allergy Clin Immunol* 2002;**109**:162–70.

8   Kay AB (ed). Hymenoptera hypersensitivity. Position paper on allergen immunotherapy. Report of a BSACI working party. *Clin Exp Allergy* 1993;**23**(Suppl 3):11–13.

9   McHugh SM, Deighton J, Stewart AG, Lachmann, PJ, Ewan PW. Bee venom immunotherapy induces a shift in cytokine responses from a TH2 to a TH1 dominant pattern: comparison of rush and conventional therapy. *Clin Exp Allergy* 1995;**25**:828–38.

10 Nasser SMS, Ying S, Meng Q, Kay AB, Ewan PW. Interleukin-10 levels increase in cutaneous biopsies of patients undergoing wasp venom immunotherapy. *Eur J Immunol* 2001;**31**:3704–13.

11 Ewan PW. New insight into immunological mechanisms of venom immunotherapy. *Curr Opinion Allergy Immunol* 2001;**1**:367–74.

Anaphylaxis

Definition

Anaphylaxis means a severe systemic allergic reaction. No universally accepted definition exists because anaphylaxis comprises a constellation of features, not all of which need to be present. A good working definition is that it involves at least one of the two severe features: respiratory difficulty (which may be due to laryngeal oedema or asthma) and hypotension (which can present as fainting, collapse or loss of consciousness). Some of the other features, especially the cutaneous features, are usually present (Box 8.3). Patients who have suffered an anaphylactic reaction should be referred to a major allergy unit.[1]

Box 8.3   Features of anaphylaxis
▶ Erythema
▶ Pruritus (generalised)
▶ Urticaria
▶ Angioedema
▶ Laryngeal oedema
▶ Asthma
▶ Rhinitis
▶ Conjunctivitis
▶ Itching of palate or external auditory meatus
▶ Palpitations
▶ Sense of impending doom
▶ Fainting, light-headedness
▶ Collapse
▶ Loss of consciousness

Clinical features

It is important to recognise that the picture will vary with the cause. When an allergen is injected systemically (as in insect stings, intravenous drugs), cardiovascular problems, especially hypotension and shock, predominate. This is especially true when large boluses are given intravenously, as at induction of anaesthesia. Foods that are absorbed transmucosally (from the oral and pharyngeal mucosa as well as the gastrointestinal tract) seem especially to cause lip, facial and laryngeal oedema. Respiratory difficulty therefore predominates in food allergy, and severe reactions are often mistaken as acute severe asthma. A key feature is the rapid onset and progression to life-threatening reactions.

Mechanism

An anaphylactic reaction results from sudden and substantial release of mast cell mediators. Classically this is IgE-mediated. Interaction of allergen with its specific IgE antibody bound to the high affinity Fcε receptors on mast cells leads to mast cell activation and mediator release.

Mast cells can be activated and release the same mediators, without the involvement of IgE antibodies. This was previously described as an anaphylactoid reaction. For clinical purposes the distinction is irrelevant as the clinical features in both anaphylactic and anaphylactoid reactions may be identical. The difference is relevant only when investigations are being considered.

Recommendations from the European Academy of Allergy and Clinical Immunology on nomenclature suggest that all reactions should now be called anaphylaxis.

Incidence

There are few data on the overall incidence of anaphylaxis. Data tend to focus on anaphylaxis due to a specific cause, eg allergy to penicillin or to anaesthetic drugs. However, there is considerable under-reporting, and a further problem is that anaphylaxis is often not recognised. Many fatal anaphylactic reactions are recorded as acute severe asthma. A retrospective study of anaphylaxis presenting to an A&E department found that approximately one in 3,500 patients per annum developed anaphylaxis in the community.[2] This study was retrospective and only identified reactions at the severest end of the spectrum, and will therefore underestimate the true incidence. In addition, it only identified anaphylaxis arising in the community and therefore excluded anaphylaxis arising in hospital, eg due to intravenous drugs. There is a strong clinical impression that the incidence of anaphylaxis is increasing. The number of hospital admissions (only a proportion of all cases) due to anaphylaxis doubled between 1991 and 1994 and increased seven-fold in the last decade.[3]

Aetiology

Foods, particularly peanuts, are the most common cause of anaphylaxis, and drug allergy, although greatly under-reported, is an increasing cause (see Boxes 8.4 and 8.5).[4,5] Food allergy is the most common cause of anaphylaxis in children. The most common foods to cause anaphylaxis include peanuts, tree nuts, fish, shellfish, egg and milk.

Box 8.4	Common causes of anaphylaxis

▶ Foods
▶ Bee and wasp stings
▶ Drugs
▶ Latex rubber

Box 8.5	Drugs causing anaphylaxis or anaphylactoid reactions

▶ Antibiotics (especially penicillin)
▶ Intravenous anaesthetic drugs
▶ Aspirin
▶ Non-steroidal anti-inflammatory drugs
▶ ACE inhibitors
▶ Intravenous contrast media
▶ Opioid analgesics
▶ Plasma expanders

ACE = angiotensin-converting enzyme.

A new problem which developed in the 1980s and 1990s is allergy to latex rubber. This is related to the increase in the use of latex rubber gloves by medical and paramedical staff, as well as to the increase in atopy. Rare causes include exercise, vaccines and semen. Allergen immunotherapy (desensitisation) may induce anaphylaxis (see Immunotherapy, p 80).

Investigations

The only immediate test that is useful at the time of reaction is measurement of mast cell tryptase. This is an indicator of mast cell activation but does not distinguish mechanisms or throw light on causes. Mast cell tryptase is usually, but not always, raised in severe reactions but may not be in less severe systemic reactions. It is only raised transiently so blood should ideally be taken within an hour of the onset of the reaction. In severe reactions, the tryptase may remain elevated for several hours but may be normal by four hours, so samples taken too late can miss the rise.

Management

Adrenaline (epinephrine) is the most important drug for anaphylaxis and should be given intramuscularly.[6,7] It is almost always effective, particularly if given soon after the onset of severe symptoms.

This should be followed by chlorpheniramine and hydrocortisone (intramuscular or slow intravenous injection). This is usually all that is required provided that treatment is started early. Treatment failure is more likely if administration of adrenaline is delayed. Biphasic reactions have been described but are probably rare; administration of hydrocortisone should minimise the risk of late relapse.

Diagnosis

Patients who have had an anaphylactic reaction should be referred to an allergist so that aetiology can be determined. The first step is to take a detailed history. In the case of an IgE-mediated reaction, the cause can usually be confirmed by demonstrating specific IgE antibodies by skin prick test or in the serum by RAST test. There are no simple diagnostic tests to confirm non-IgE-mediated anaphylactic reactions. These are sometimes clear from the history, eg a reaction after taking aspirin, but sometimes confirmation is only possible if a challenge test is performed, eg this may be required where several drugs known to cause non-IgE reactions were taken together. Graded doses of the suspect cause, eg a drug, are given. This carries the risk of inducing anaphylaxis and should only be done in a specialist allergy unit, by those with experience in treating anaphylaxis.

Further management

Avoidance of the cause is a key part of management and should be implemented. If there is a risk of further reactions (eg if avoidance is difficult), it is usually appropriate to provide an adrenaline auto-injector, with a written treatment plan and appropriate training.

In the case of children, provision of adrenaline auto-injectors such as Epipen® for emergency use means that parents, carers and school staff need to be trained. A system to implement training of school staff was pioneered in Cambridge and has now been adopted in other parts of the country.[8] However, lack of allergy services means that it is often not possible to be referred to an appropriate specialist, and that there are no trained community paediatric units to provide training for school staff.

Implementation of this type of management plan has been shown to be effective in nut allergy in reducing the incidence and severity of further reactions.[9] In a series of 567 patients with nut allergy, only 15% had further reaction (compared to an expected 50% if patients tried to avoid nuts but did not have professional advice) and most of these were mild, requiring no treatment or an oral antihistamine. A further reaction requiring adrenaline was rare, but self-treatment was always effective.

References

1 Department of Health. *National specialised services definitions set.* Specialised services for allergy, definition no 17 (all ages). DH website: www.doh.gov.uk

2 Stewart AG, Ewan PW. The incidence, aetiology and management of anaphylaxis presenting to an Accident & Emergency department. *QJM* 1996;**89**:859–64.

3 Sheikh A, Alves B. Hospital admissions for acute anaphylaxis: time trend study. *BMJ* 2000;**320**:1441.

4 Tariq SM, Stevens M, Matthews W, Ridout S *et al.* Cohort study of peanut and tree nut sensitisation by age of 4 years. *BMJ* 1996;**313**:514–7.

5 Grundy J, Matthews S, Bateman B, Dean T, Arshad SH. Rising prevalence of allergy to peanut in children: data from 2 sequential cohorts. *J Allergy Clin Immunol* 2002;**110**:784–9.

6 Project Team of the UK Resuscitation Council. The emergency medical treatment of anaphylactic reactions. *J Accid Emerg Med* 1999;**16**:243–7.

7 Ewan PW. Treatment of anaphylactic reactions. *Prescribers' Journal* 1997;**37**:125–32.

8   Vickers DW, Maynard L, Ewan PW. Management of children with potential anaphylactic reactions in the community: a training package and proposals for good practice. *Clin Exp Allergy* 1997;27:898–903.

9   Ewan PW, Clark AT. Long-term prospective observational study of the outcome of a management plan in patients with peanut and nut allergy referred to a regional allergy centre. *Lancet* 2001;357:111–15.

Occupational allergy

Almost all the adult allergic diseases can arise from exposures encountered at work, the most common being allergic skin rashes, rhinitis and asthma. Although sometimes originating from exposures outside work, allergy-related symptoms can be exacerbated by irritant agents at work. To complicate matters further, people with allergies may be barred from some occupations and find others particularly difficult to sustain. These issues are likely to become increasingly prominent, given the increasing prevalence of many allergic diseases in the UK.

The most common allergic diseases caused by occupational exposures are:

1   Contact *dermatitis*, arising from a delayed-type immunological response to one or more of a large number of occupational exposures, especially amines, epoxy resins, metals (eg nickel), fragrances and halogenated compounds. This condition accounts for around half of all days lost from work through sickness.[1]

2   A protein *dermatitis*, urticarial in character, arising from an immediate-type hypersensitivity and associated with IgE antibody production against a biological allergen encountered at work.

3   Occupational *asthma* which is often accompanied by:

4   Occupational *rhinitis* and *allergic eye disease* (conjunctivitis) The mechanisms of occupational nasal and eye allergies are analogous to those that give rise to occupational asthma and in most cases they are characterised by the production of specific IgE antibodies against the offending agent(s).

5   Occupational allergies occasionally may present with *anaphylaxis*.

As with other allergic diseases, it is clear that occupational allergies may present to a variety of clinical specialists and with a variety of symptoms. In general, they are clinically indistinct from non-occupational allergies and from non-allergic 'irritant' reactions. The origin of a workplace allergy will only be identified if there is sufficient and widespread awareness that occupational diseases are not uncommon. At present, there is good evidence that this is not the case and that as a consequence a high proportion of occupational disease is missed. This is important since these are usually preventable diseases; at an individual level, treatment or cure is rarely possible unless the occupational agent causing the disease is recognised.

Occupational allergies generally have a clear temporal relationship with a particular type of work or workplace; ie they begin shortly after starting a new job – or a change in exposure within a job – and, importantly, they tend to improve away from work. The clinical history of the disease is all important in diagnosis, as is a detailed knowledge of occupational processes and exposures. Investigations are similar to those for other allergic diseases but access to the necessary test reagents is very limited. Similarly, the interpretation of test results is not necessarily straightforward and frequently requires specialist expertise. Because the implications of an occupational allergy are socially, economically and often legally important, it is helpful if the clinician is also experienced in these areas.

In the UK, there are nation-wide surveillance schemes which record the annual incidence of occupational skin and respiratory diseases ('EPIDERM'* and 'SWORD' respectively). These are, however, limited to reports from specialist physicians and they do not record disease which is managed entirely within primary care or disease which never reaches medical attention. In addition, much occupational allergy is identified and managed within the occupational health services. Nevertheless, it is of concern that there is no evidence in the UK that any of the occupational allergic diseases, which are largely preventable, are diminishing in frequency.[2]

Occupational asthma

The issue of occupational allergy and its impact on society is exemplified by the particular case of occupational asthma. In the UK and across western Europe and North America, about 10% of adult asthma is attributable to workplace exposures.[3] This figure is derived from meta-analysis of epidemiological studies and it is unclear what proportion represents *de novo* sensitisation to workplace allergens (ie true 'occupational asthma'). In all probability most asthma is constitutional, provoked or exacerbated by irritant exposures at work ('work-related' asthma). True occupational asthma, which is initiated by one or more exposures at work, is probably less common but remains an important medical, social and industrial issue. With 1,200 new cases each year in the UK, it is the most common occupational lung disease reported to SWORD.[2] There is no doubt that this figure is a considerable underestimate of the true incidence.[4,5] The average age at diagnosis is 43 years, with about 75% of reported cases occurring in men. The incidence of occupational rhinitis and eye symptoms, which frequently accompany asthma, is unmeasured but they are probably more common than workplace asthma itself.

Over 300 workplace agents have been identified as causing asthma. However, only a dozen of these are responsible for three-quarters of the occupational asthma recognised in the UK. Among these are the diisocyanates, highly reactive chemicals which are used widely in industry and are apparently the most common single agent giving rise to occupational asthma. Laboratory animal proteins, flour, a wide variety of enzymes, latex and electronic solder fume are other important agents. Table 8.3 summarises 'high-risk' occupations in the UK.

In most cases, occupational asthma is clinically indistinguishable from the more classical allergic forms of the disease. However, even with treatment it does not improve unless all (workplace) exposure to the causative agent is prevented, which usually requires a change of occupation. The social and economic consequences of occupational and work-related asthma are significant, and are certainly greater than those accompanying other forms of the disease.[6]

The distinction between work-related and occupational asthma is important for functional, prognostic, therapeutic, socio-economic and legal reasons. It is often a distinction which requires specialist investigation.[7] There are six specialist respiratory centres in the UK which specialise in the management of occupational asthma, several concentrating largely on medico-legal cases. Two centres are responsible for most newly reported cases. A substantial proportion of the

---

*EPIDERM: Centre for Occupational and Environmental Health, Stopford Building, Oxford Road, Manchester M13 9PT.

Table 8.3   High-risk occupations in the UK

'High molecular weight' agents		'Low molecular weight' agents	
Occupation	Agent(s)	Occupation	Agent(s)
Baker	Flour(s) Enzymes Egg-white	Spray painter	Hexamethylene Diisocyanate
Laboratory animal worker	Animal proteins Latex	Plastics/foam manufacturer	Toluene diisocyanate
Healthcare worker	Latex	Other industry	Methylene diphenyldiisocyanate
Detergent manufacturer	Detergent enzymes	Electronic solderer	Colophony fume
Tea packer	Herbal tea dusts	Circuit board manufacturer	Colophony fume Cyanoacrylate Persulphates
Seafood processor	Fish and crustacean proteins	Resin/paint manufacturer	Acid anyhdrides
Factory workers	Latex	Precious metal refiner	Platinum salts
		Hairdresser	Persulphates

disease (about 25%), is diagnosed and managed within the occupational health service; these cases tend to be recognised earlier and are less severe than those reported by chest physicians.[4]

Latex allergy

This is important in those who wear rubber gloves, particularly healthcare workers and laboratory workers. The prevalence has risen substantially with the increased use of surgical gloves. Whereas there were only two case reports by 1979, a recent study showed that 16% of healthcare workers were sensitised (ie had positive tests for latex-specific IgE antibodies), and that about half of these had clinical reactions on exposure to latex rubber.

References

1   Wilkinson JD, Shaw S, Kay B (ed). *Contact dermatitis in allergy and allergic diseases.* Oxford: Blackwell, 1997.

2   McDonald JC, Keynes HL, Meredith SK. Reported incidence of occupational asthma in the United Kingdom, 1989–1997. *Occup Environ Med* 2000;**57**:823–9.

3   Blanc PD, Toren K. How much adult asthma can be attributed to occupational factors? *Am J Med* 1999;**107**:580–7.

4   Ross DJ. Ten years of the SWORD project. *Clin Exp Allergy* 1999;**29**:750–3.

5   Draper A, Cullinan P, Newman Taylor AJ. Laboratory animal workers in the UK; estimating the denominator. *Occup Environ Med* 2003 (in press).

6   Cannon J, Cullinan P, Newman Taylor AJ. Consequences of occupational asthma. *BMJ* 1995;**311**:602–3.

7   Newman Taylor AJ, Cullinan P. Diagnosis of occupational lung disease. In: Mapp CE (ed) *Occupational lung disorders. European Respiratory Monograph* 1999;**11**:64–105.

9. Diagnostic tests

Skin prick or laboratory tests can help to confirm the clinical diagnosis in allergy. However, these tests are of limited value without a detailed clinical history.

Simple allergies such as hay fever do not require confirmatory diagnostic tests (the exception being when immunotherapy is to be given). In other conditions it is essential to demonstrate specific IgE antibody, and this can be done by a skin prick test (SPT) or by measuring specific IgE in the serum. These are different ways of measuring the same antibody response, but the SPT is superior. Confirmation of the diagnosis is required: in any severe allergy; where avoidance measures will be instituted (eg for house dust mite, food, drug or latex allergy); if immunotherapy is required; and in other conditions if the diagnosis is not clear from the history.

Suspected allergens can also be injected directly into the skin (intradermal (ID) tests), but they can produce painful reactions, are technically more difficult, and sometimes give misleading results because the needle itself can cause sufficient damage to produce a false-positive response.

The measurement of allergen-specific IgE in serum has improved markedly over the last decade. Specific IgE against a wide range of well validated allergens is now available. Measurement of allergen-specific IgE is of value when facilities for SPT are unavailable or when SPT is otherwise contradicted, eg atopic dermatitis involving areas where SPTs are performed, or in patients taking H_1-antihistamine. However, for other allergens, serum-specific IgE tests are either (i) not available, or (ii) available but of poor quality, eg fruits and vegetables, and for some of these SPTs can be performed using the prick–prick test technique.

Special challenge (provocation) tests may be needed to make the diagnosis of allergy, for example to foods and drugs, when often there are no validated skin tests or laboratory tests and/or the mechanism does not involve IgE. Double-blind placebo-controlled tests can often identify or disprove food intolerance by giving suspected foods or food additives in disguised forms. Allergen inhalation tests can confirm suspected causes of occupational asthma.

SPTs are cheap and easy to perform once staff are trained, whereas serum IgE tests are more costly but still relatively cheap. Challenge tests are a day-case procedure in a specialist allergy unit with facilities and expertise for treating anaphylaxis. Patch testing for contact dermatitis is valuable and is done primarily in dermatology departments. Lymphocyte transformation tests and basophil histamine release or flow cytometry analysis of cell surface 'activation' markers have been reported to be helpful for diagnosing drug allergies, but these tests have not yet been validated. An appraisal of the currently available clinical and laboratory tests in use is displayed in Table 9.1. Tests of no proven value are shown in Table 9.2. In all cases the tests should be used to support clinical history and investigation.

Table 9.1	Tests used in allergy diagnosis			
Test	**How is test performed?**	**Rationale**	**Indication**	**Interpretation/limitations**
Skin prick test (SPT)	Rapid *in vivo* test, normally performed on forearm using standardised commercial liquid extracts lightly pricked into the epidermis. Inexpensive and can be read after a short interval.	Detects specific IgE bound to mast cells. Allergen reacts with specific IgE antibodies on skin mast cells producing a wheal and flare at the site, if positive.	Testing against pollens, animal dander, house dust mite, moulds, insect venom, foods, latex and certain drugs.	Must be interpreted in context of clinical history as positive results reveal sensitivity not necessarily symptomatic allergy. Positive and negative controls are essential.
Intradermal testing	As for SPTs but requires a higher level of technical expertise to inject allergen solution into the dermis.	Detects specific IgE bound to mast cells. More allergen injected. Larger oedematous reaction.	Now that potent extracts are available for SPTs, intradermal testing has few clinical advantages and can be associated with adverse reactions.	Widely used in North America as an alternative to SPTs, but Europe favours SPTs.
Total serum IgE	Total serum IgE antibodies are measured in the laboratory.	IgE antibodies are involved in immediate allergy, but allergen-specific IgE is far more clinically relevant.	Useful in interpreting specific IgE tests measured in blood.	In isolation, a total serum IgE does not have diagnostic value but should stimulate further investigations.
Allergen-specific IgE	Allergen-specific IgE antibodies in serum bind to immobilised allergen. The traditional RAST has been replaced by immunoassays namely ELISA.	Identification of allergen-specific IgE in the laboratory.	Can be used as a substitute for SPTs but is expensive and results are usually not rapidly available.	Interpret in the light of the clinical history. Low values must be interpreted with caution especially if the total serum IgE is high.
Challenge tests	Double-blind placebo-controlled food challenge (DBPCFC) involves giving a concealed test food where the subject and the test supervisor are unaware which is the adulterated dish.	To confirm or refute adverse food reactions whilst minimising extraneous influences.	When specific IgE not available or not involved. Where there is a discrepancy between the clinical history and specific IgE by SPTs and/or blood tests. To determine resolution of allergy.	DBPCFCs are extremely time consuming although remain the gold standard for the diagnosis of adverse food reactions. Open challenges are notorious for their misleading results.
Patch testing	A standard battery of non-irritating allergens is applied to healthy skin (usually the back) under an occlusive dressing. The tests are usually read at 48 and 72 hours.	Sensitised white blood cells (T lymphocytes) traffic to the skin in contact with the allergen to produce local inflammation.	Used in the diagnosis of allergic contact dermatitis to substances such as nickel, dyes and latex. Performed in dermatology departments.	Must be read by an experienced physician and interpretation can be problematical as no positive control is possible.

Table 9.1	Tests used in allergy diagnosis – *continued*			
Test	**How is test performed?**	**Rationale**	**Indication**	**Interpretation/limitations**
Serum tryptase	Measured on blood using standard laboratory technologies.	Mast cell activation releases tryptase. This occurs through IgE and non-IgE mechanisms.	Investigation of collapse or suspected allergic reactions especially anaesthetic-induced reactions. Shows the reaction was due to mast cell activation.	Only high levels are significant and samples must be taken during the reaction or in the period immediately following the reaction.
Basophil activation tests and histamine release assays	White cells are isolated from peripheral blood and exposed to soluble allergens that react to IgE molecules on their surface.	If allergen-specific IgE is present on these cells then they will develop a certain surface marker (CD63) and will release histamine.	Either histamine release or CD63 expression can be of value in identifying certain drug reactions. Available mainly on a research basis.	These are expensive and demanding laboratory assays, presently used primarily as research tools. Expensive equipment is required for CD63 measurement.
Atopy patch test (APT)	Allergen extracts are applied to uninvolved abraded skin, under cups for 48 hours, then read at successive intervals. Positive reactions are denoted by redness and occasional small blisters.	Allergen-specific testing of mostly non-IgE-mediated skin reactions.	APT may help in the diagnosis of food allergy in children with atopic dermatitis, when the history suggests a possible late-phase reaction related to food.	Problems include standardisation and concentration of extracts used. Its clinical role is still being evaluated.
Lymphocyte transformation test	Isolated peripheral blood white cells (T lymphocytes) are reacted with a given allergen, usually a drug, and the proliferative response measured.	Cell-mediated immune responses may underlie certain drug allergies.	Reported to be useful in certain penicillin allergies. Used mainly on a research basis.	The test is time consuming, labour intensive and expensive. Lack of standards makes interpretation difficult without controls.

ELISA = enzyme-linked immunosorbent assay.

Table 9.2	Alternative tests of no proven value in allergy diagnosis			
Test	**How is test performed?**	**Rationale**	**Indication**	**Interpretation/limitations**
Electrodermal testing – Vegatest	Small changes in skin electrical resistance in response to test substances placed in a low voltage electrical circuit.	Small changes in resistance are used to assess sensitivity to potential allergens.	No validated use. Used to assess an individual's allergic status to foods and inhaled allergens.	Although commonly used in the UK, electrodermal testing cannot be recommended for the diagnosis of environmental allergies.[1,2]
Food specific IgG antibodies	Food specific IgG antibodies are measured by immunoassay (ELISA). A finger prick blood sample on absorbent wand is the usual format.	Specific IgG antibodies are suggested to identify food sensitive individuals. The role of these IgG antibodies in the pathogenesis of these conditions is not established.	No validated use. Used for possible food sensitivity related to chronic disease.	Dietary advice including food avoidance and food rotation is made depending on result. However, these antibodies are present in normal healthy subjects. Randomised control trials to establish the value of IgG antibodies in food sensitivity are required.
Hair analysis	Hair sample from near the scalp.	Mineral analysis is undertaken in private laboratories using techniques that are not validated or controlled against standard materials.	No validated use. Claims to determine the person's health and nutritional, vitamin and mineral status.	No evidence that low concentration of an element in a hair sample reflects low body stores. Mineral content of hair is affected by age, gender and geographical location, and exposure to dyes and bleaches.[3]
Cytotoxic food testing – leuco-cytotoxic test	A drop of diluted whole blood is placed on a slide pre-coated with a food extract and studied under the microscope after an interval.	Distortion or swelling of the white blood cells is said to indicate food allergy.	No validated use. Claims to identify food sensitivities causing a variety of medical conditions including asthma, eczema, hypertension and fatigue.	A number of controlled trials have indicated that leucocytotoxic testing is ineffective for the diagnosis of food and inhalant allergy.[4]
NuTron test	Whole peripheral blood is incubated with in-house pure solutions of food. The sample is then processed in an automated haematology analyser to measure neutrophil activation.	Certain foods pass through the gut into the circulation leading to chemical reactions and inflammation.	No validated use. Promotional material recommends this test for food intolerance and problems with candida.	No validation or research evidence to support these claims.

Table 9.2   Alternative tests of no proven value in allergy diagnosis – *continued*

Test	How is test performed?	Rationale	Indication	Interpretation/limitations
Iris diagnosis – iridology	Close examination of the iris of the eye.	The belief is that an area of the iris represents each area of the body. A naturopath developed this idea 70 years ago.	No validated use. Theory is that a person's state of health and disease can be diagnosed from the colour, texture, and location of various pigment flecks on the iris.	Advice on treatment with herbs, vitamins and minerals is given. There is no scientific basis or validation for these claims.
Pulse test	The pulse is taken, test food consumed and the pulse re-recorded.	Allergy causes a change in pulse. An increase of ≥10 beats/min is deemed 'diagnostic'.	No validated use. Used in food allergy.	Unproven and likely to be influenced by the patient's state of anxiety etc.

ELISA = enzyme-linked immunosorbent assay.

1   Lewith GT, Kenyon JN, Broomfield J, Prescott P *et al*. Is electrodermal testing as effective as skin prick tests for diagnosing allergies? A double blind, randomised block design study. *BMJ* 2001;**332**:131–4.

2   Semizzi M, Senna G, Crivellaro M, Rapacioli G *et al*. A double-blind, placebo-controlled study on the diagnostic accuracy of an electrodermal test in allergic subjects. *Clin Exp Allergy* 2002;**32**(6):928–32.

3   KM Hambidge. Hair analyses: worthless for vitamins, limited for minerals. *Am J Clin Nutr* 1982;**36**:943–9.

4   American Academy of Allergy: position statements – controversial techniques. *J Allergy Clin Immunol* 1981;**67**(5):333–8.

10. Specialist services: treatment and challenge tests

The basic principles in the treatment of allergic diseases are:

(i) identification and avoidance of allergic triggers

(ii) effective use of drugs, avoiding side effects where possible

(iii) use of immunotherapy (desensitisation), where appropriate.

Identification of allergic and non-allergic triggers is an essential part of diagnosis. Wherever practical, allergen avoidance should be considered as the first line of treatment (see Chapter 7, pp 35–40). In some cases, particularly in mono-allergy, this can completely abrogate symptoms, eg in drug, food or animal allergy. For other allergens, such as house dust mite or pollens, reducing the allergen load can reduce symptoms or allow better control with the same drug, or a lower dose of it.[1] Recognition of allergens that cause severe seasonal symptoms, eg *Alternaria*-induced asthma, allows the introduction of prophylactic therapy before allergen exposure, and prevention of exacerbations and hospital admission.

This chapter describes some areas of treatment best provided by specialist allergists; for treatments for allergic reactions to specific foods and drugs, see Chapter 8. Specialist services suitable for regional commissioning have been defined by the Department of Health.[2] Outlines of treatments for specific allergic diseases are given in Chapter 8.

Anaphylaxis

The cause should be identified and advice on avoidance given. The key drug for the acute attack is adrenaline administered intramuscularly.[3,4] This is usually followed by injected chlorpheniramine and hydrocortisone. If there is a likelihood of further attacks, for example if avoidance is difficult, patients are given written self-held treatment plans and emergency medication. Selection of the appropriate drugs is important because early treatment is vital and can be life-saving. Also required are training in recognition of reactions, in self- or parent-administration of drugs, and training of school staff if a child is involved.[5,6]

Glottal oedema

Ideally the cause, eg a drug, should be identified and avoided. However, this is not always possible, and additionally a proportion of patients have idiopathic glottal oedema, so attacks may recur. Medical treatment of acute attacks depends on the severity, but relies on early administration. An allergist can provide patients with a written treatment plan and drugs for self-administration. These include high dose oral antihistamines, oral steroids, topical adrenaline from an inhaler or intramuscular adrenaline.

Immunotherapy (desensitisation)

Specific immunotherapy switches off responses to allergen, and is thus a different approach from drug therapy.[7]

Efficacy

Controlled studies have shown that immunotherapy is effective in seasonal allergic rhinitis, mild allergic asthma, and allergy to bee and wasp stings.[8,9,10] Successful controlled trials with cat dander and the house dust mite, and in perennial allergic rhinitis, have been reported but more studies are needed. Immunotherapy is of no value in non-allergic rhinitis, atopic dermatitis, chronic urticaria, or food hypersensitivity.

Indications

In UK practice, immunotherapy is the first line of treatment in allergy to wasp and bee venom, and in severe summer hay fever that has failed to respond to anti-allergic drugs.[7,11] Because immunotherapy is relatively expensive and requires considerable commitment from both doctor and patient, the cost/benefit ratio should be assessed in each case. Immunotherapy is currently not recommended in the UK for patients with chronic asthma because this is less likely to respond and side effects are much more frequent.

Practical aspects

Immunotherapy consists of subcutaneous injections of extracts of the relevant allergens, given in increasing amounts (during the initial course) until the top dose is reached. Treatment is continued, repeating the maintenance dose, usually for three years. Benefits last for several years after completing the course of injections. Allergenic extracts must be carefully prepared, standardised and of adequate potency.

The safety of immunotherapy must be considered, particularly because of its ability to cause systemic allergic reactions. The incidence of systemic anaphylactic responses to immuno-therapy is increased in rhinitis patients with co-existent asthma. Although more common in the initial course, severe systemic reactions can occur at any time during the three-year course. Monitoring is important and patients are observed carefully for one hour after each injection, as severe reactions occur in this period.

For these reasons, immunotherapy should be conducted in allergy centres by allergists who are experienced in its use, who know when to modify treatment protocols, who can recognise reactions early and are experienced in treating anaphylaxis. Drugs for treatment of anaphylaxis and acute asthma must be immediately available. Patient selection is also important. Immunotherapy requires a team approach, with allergy specialist nurses as well as doctors, and is best concentrated in centres treating large numbers of patients.

Mechanism

The mechanism of action is thought to involve induction of T-cell tolerance, either by shifting the balance of T-cell cytokine production or by inducing allergen-specific regulatory T-cells with enhanced IL-10 secretion and production of allergen-specific protective IgG4 anti-bodies.[12,13] Early in immunotherapy, there is no reduction in allergen-specific IgE concentrations or in immediate skin test responses, but in the late phase, response to allergen is almost abolished.[14] In the maintenance phase, serum IgE antibody concentrations and immediate skin test responses begin to decline. There is evidence of downregulation of effector cells including eosinophils and basophils.[15–17] In practice, patients who receive specific immunotherapy are protected from the effects of natural exposure to allergen, and show a reduction in sensitivity of target organs (eg nose, eyes or lower airways).

Other vaccines

For many years there has been interest in administering desensitising vaccines in low doses and by routes other than subcutaneous injections, ie by the oral, inhaled or sublingual routes. Further studies are required to establish efficacy and safety.

Future therapies

Vaccines using modified allergens are currently being developed to treat peanut allergy, but they require rigorous evaluation for both efficacy and safety before being introduced into clinical practice.

Future research is likely to produce more effective and safer forms of specific immunotherapy, and there will probably be new immunomodulatory treatments, exploiting recent discoveries on the actions and regulation of cytokines, interleukins and chemokines etc, which regulate IgE, cellular recruitment and the downstream consequences of allergic reactions. A blocking monoclonal antibody against IgE (eg omalizumab), when administered by subcutaneous injection at 2–4 week intervals, is highly effective in allergic asthma, rhinitis, and peanut allergy, and may soon be available for treating the more severe forms of this disease.[18–21] Clinical trials are in progress to assess the efficacy and safety of agents that enhance 'innate' (as opposed to adaptive) immunity, eg extracts of mycobacteria and bacterial DNA sequences (CpG), either alone or in combination with specific immunotherapy.

Challenge tests

Challenge tests are important in allergy diagnosis and are performed in major allergy centres.[2] They are required when there is no other way of confirming or refuting a possible cause of a reaction. This occurs when there is no diagnostic test, or where several putative causes occur simultaneously, mostly in the case of drugs and foods. Challenge tests are required in suspected local anaesthetic allergy, and are often used for non-steroidal anti-inflammatory drugs/aspirin or antibiotics. They can also be used to show that allergy has resolved, eg a food allergy, or whether patients who are sensitised (positive specific IgE) without known exposure are or are not clinically allergic.

Incremental doses of the test substance are given at intervals, until a systemic reaction occurs or the full dose is tolerated. Monitoring is essential, and treatment for all grades of allergic reaction, including anaphylaxis, must be available.

References

1   Custovic A, Murray CS, Gore RB, Woodcock A. Environmental allergen control. *Ann Allergy Asthma Immunol* 2002;**88**:432–41.

2   Department of Health. *National specialised services definitions set.* Specialist services for Allergy, Definition no. 17 (all ages). DH website: www.doh.gov.uk

3   Project team of the UK Rescuscitation Council. The emergency medical treatment of anaphylactic reactions. *J Accid Emerg Med* 1999;**16**:243–7.

4   Ewan PW. Treatment of anaphylactic reactions. *Prescribers Journal* 1997;**37**:125–32.

5   Ewan PW, Clark AT. Long term prospective observational study of the outcome of a management plan in patients with peanut and nut allergy referred to a regional allergy centre. *Lancet* 2001;**356**:111–?14.

6   Vickers DW, Maynard L, Ewan PW. Management of children with potential anaphylactic reactions in the community: a training package and proposals for good practice. *Clin Exp Allergy* 1997;**27**:898–903.

7   Varga EM, Durham SR. Allergen injection immunotherapy. *Clin Allergy Immunol* 2002;**16**:533–49.

8   Walker SM, Varney VA, Gaga M, Jacobson MR, Durham SR. Grass pollen immunotherapy: efficacy and safety during a 4-year follow-up study. *Allergy* 1995;**50**(5):405–13.

9   Walker SM, Pajno GB, Lima MT, Wilson DR, Durham SR. Grass pollen immunotherapy for seasonal rhinitis and asthma: a randomized, controlled trial. *J Allergy Clin Immunol* 2001;**107**(1):87–93.

10 Durham SR, Walker SM, Varga EM, Jacobson MR *et al.* Long-term clinical efficacy of grass-pollen immunotherapy. *N Engl J Med* 1999;**341**(7):468–75.

11 Kay AB (ed). Position paper on allergen immunotherapy: report of a BSACI working party. *Clin Exp Allergy* 1993;suppl 3.

12 Durham SR, Ying S, Varney VA, Jacobson M *et al.* Grass pollen immunotherapy inhibits allergen-induced infiltration of CD4+ T lymphocytes and eosinophils in the nasal mucosa and increases the number of cells expressing messenger RNA for interferon-gamma. *J Allergy Clin Immunol* 1996;**97**(6):1356–65.

13 Nasser SMS, Ying S, Meng Q, Kay AB, Ewan PW. Interleukin-10 levels increase in cutaneous biopsies of patients undergoing wasp venom immunotherapy. *Eur J Immunol* 2001;**31**:3704–13.

14 Varney VA, Hamid QA, Gaga M, Ying S *et al.* Influence of grass pollen immunotherapy on cellular infiltration and cytokine mRNA expression during allergen-induced late-phase cutaneous responses. *J Clin Invest* 1993;**92**(2):644–51.

15 Wilson DR, Nouri-Aria KT, Walker SM, Pajno GB *et al.* Grass pollen immunotherapy: symptomatic improvement correlates with reductions in eosinophils and IL-5 mRNA expression in the nasal mucosa during the pollen season. *J Allergy Clin Immunol* 2001;**107**(6):971–6.

16 Wilson DR, Irani AM, Walker SM, Jacobson MR *et al.* Grass pollen immunotherapy inhibits seasonal increases in basophils and eosinophils in the nasal epithelium. *Clin Exp Allergy* 2001;**31**(11):1705–13.

17 Durham SR, Varney VA, Gaga M, Jacobson MR *et al.* Grass pollen immunotherapy decreases the number of mast cells in the skin. *Clin Exp Allergy* 1999;**29**(11):1490–6.

18 Soler M, Matz J, Townley R, Buhl R *et al.* The anti-IgE antibody omalizumab reduces exacerbations and steroid requirement in allergic asthmatics. *Eur Respir J* 2001;**18**(2):254–61.

19 Babu KS, Arshad SH, Holgate ST. Omalizumab, a novel anti-IgE therapy in allergic disorders. *Expert Opin Biol Ther* 2001;**1**(6):1049–58.

20 Corren J, Casale T, Deniz Y, Ashby M. Omalizumab, a recombinant humanized anti-IgE antibody, reduces asthma-related emergency room visits and hospitalizations in patients with allergic asthma. *J Allergy Clin Immunol* 2003;**111**(1):87–90.

21 Leung DYM, Sampson HA, Yuninger JW, Burkes AW *et al.* Effect of anti-IgE therapy in patients with peanut allergy. *N Engl J Med* 2003;**348**;986–93.

11. Prevention

Factors to be considered in relation to prevention of allergy include genetic susceptibility, environmental exposure, and immunotherapy.

Studies of twins indicate that both genetic and environmental factors contribute in equal measure to the development of allergy especially atopy.[1] These factors operate at one or more levels of disorder: systemic immune dysfunction, local immune dysfunction (mucosal immunity), or 'target' organ in which the allergy is expressed (eg in the lower airways, nose, skin or gut). The genetic and environmental interactions will influence primary, secondary and tertiary preventative strategies at interfaces of genetic susceptibility and immune response (primary prevention), expression of the immune response into an allergic inflammatory disorder (secondary prevention), and gradations of allergic tissue responses in specific organs (tertiary prevention).

Genetic factors

The genetic susceptibility to develop allergy and its organ-specific expression involves many genes that interact with each other and the environment. Use of gene markers spaced at intervals across all of the chromosomes (linkage studies) indicates multiple chromosomal regions that are linked to distinct immune or target-organ disease expression. Although they also show the impact of racial origin,[2] some linkages cross racial groups, eg those on chromosome 5 and chromosome 12. The identification of novel disease susceptibility genes in regions of chromosomal linkage (positional cloning) are now set to reveal previously unidentified loci which contribute to atopy and its associated clinical disorders; one recently reported asthma gene is a proteolytic enzyme (ADAM 33) encoded on chromosome 20.[3]

Candidate gene studies, some allied to the linkage data, are already yeilding more precise information. For example, common genetic variants of Th-2 immune signalling (eg IL-4, IL-13 and their receptors and cell signalling machinery) are significant risk factors for atopy (systemic immunity) and asthma (local mucosal immunity).[4] Also, asthma phenotypes and responses to therapy (long-acting bronchodilator β_2-adrenergic agonists) are associated with certain genetic variants of the β_2-adrenergic receptor.[5]

Rapid genetic assays and the systematic collection of large populations will permit more precise definition of which genes interact at different locations. It should then be possible to predict risk of atopic immune disorders and the different clinical syndromes. Identification of genetic risk for atopy in particular individuals, through complex DNA analysis, will be a basis for targeted environmental manipulations at different levels of prevention (see below). Clarification of the major genetic inputs will also highlight the 'pathways' that lead to atopic immune disorder and accompanying clinical disorders. This, allied to the development of specific inhibitors (eg monoclonal antibodies and specific RNA interference (RNAi))[6] of molecules in such pathways, will lead to novel strategies at the secondary and tertiary levels, and perhaps, ultimately, at the primary level of disease prevention.

Environmental factors

The importance of factors in the environment that initiate and maintain allergic disorders is emphasised by the recent increase in their prevalence. This suggests that some factor(s) associated with 'westernisation' are centrally involved.[7] Current epidemiological data provide intriguing pointers, and it is hoped that intervention trials will clarify the important preventive targets. The following areas are noteworthy.

Allergens   Allergens are the environmental targets for atopic response, and the major disease-associated allergens vary according to geographical location. Limiting exposure clearly helps in tertiary prevention, but this is not always possible:[8] for example, people who are allergic to pet allergens may still choose to keep their pets. Workers should withdraw from exposure to occupational agents. Useful house dust mite control can be achieved,[9] but the benefit derived remains to be satisfactorily clarified.[10,11]

The hygiene hypothesis   Exposure in early life to infectious agents and their products, and their potential limitation of atopic immune response, may provide a novel approach to both primary and secondary prevention.[12,13] Microbial exposures may limit atopy through the induction of Th-1 immunity (in turn suppressing Th-2 immunity through cytokine activity), or through the induction of immune regulating mechanisms involving special suppressive T lymphocytes.[14] Epidemiological studies that support the 'hygiene concept' show association between exposures to commonly found bacteria that exist in the gut of humans, mycobacteria, measles and hepatitis A in early life and less atopy.[13] In mice, mycobacterial immunisation is an effective limiter of experimental allergy.[15] Trials in humans are now needed, and investigations of microbial immunisations, by mouth or by injection, have started for both secondary and tertiary prevention of allergy.

Some studies record associations between atopy and immunisations to both pertussis and measles.[16] Thus, as the number of public health immunisations steadily climbs, their effects on immune mechanisms and atopy needs more careful monitoring because of the possibility that certain genetic subgroups may be susceptible to the promotion of atopy by vaccines. Likewise, antibiotic use in early life has been repeatedly associated with more atopy;[16] early-life administration of antibiotics increases Th-2 immune activity in mice.[17] Further study is important to exclude reverse causation and to clarify the mechanisms of action of any causal effect.[18]

Good industrial practice   Good industrial practice, for instance in the use of isocyanates and acid anhydrides which are potent causes of asthma, is vital in the primary prevention of occupational allergy.[19] Good practice can also greatly reduce problems with dermatitis.

Diet   The diet of pregnant mothers and infants in 'westernised' countries is very different from that of their counterparts in the developing world. The western diet has been considered a candidate for promoting atopy, perhaps through deficiency (eg vitamin E and other anti-oxidants caused by diets low in fruit and vegetables) or excess (eg saturated fats and protein).[20] This could become an important area for primary and secondary prevention; much further study is needed.

Chemical air pollution   This comes in many forms but the weight of evidence suggests that particulate and gaseous air pollution impinge more on the expression of disease than its causation.[21] Therefore, attempts to control such air pollution, through public measures limiting car exhaust fumes for example, may be helpful in both secondary and tertiary prevention. Recent unconfirmed epidemiological data suggest that ozone may play a role in triggering asthma.[21] This needs much further work but raises the question of whether control of outdoor air pollution from vehicle exhaust might be effective in primary prevention.

Parental smoking   *In utero* and early-life exposure to tobacco smoke are adverse factors for asthma and should be avoided, but their relationship to atopy is less clear.[22]

Breast-feeding   Although some studies show modest benefit from breast-feeding in primary and secondary prevention of atopic eczema, the evidence is inconclusive.[23]

Immunotherapy

Immunotherapy may well become valuable in primary prevention, when molecular genetic methods are available for identifying genetic risk of atopic immune disorder. Its role in secondary and tertiary prevention[24] was discussed in Chapter 10, pp 80–81.

References

1   Hanson B, McGue M, Roitman-Johnson B, Segal NL *et al.* Atopic disease and immunoglobulin E in twins reared apart and together. *Am J Hum Genet* 1991; **8**(5):873–9.

2   Ober C. Susceptibility genes in asthma and allergy. *Curr Allergy Asthma Rep* 2001;**1**(2):174–9.

3   Van Eerdewegh P, Little RD, Dupuis J, Del Mastro RG *et al.* Association of the ADAM-33 gene with asthma and bronchial hyper-responsiveness. *Nature* 2002; **418**:426–30.

4   Shirakawa I, Deichmann KA, Izuhara I, Mao I *et al.* Atopy and asthma: genetic variants of IL-4 and IL-13 signalling. *Immunol Today* 2000;**21**(2):60–4.

5   Fenech A, Hall IP. Pharmacogenetics of asthma. *Br J Clin Pharmacol* 2002;**53**(1):3–15.

6   Bass BL. RNA interference. The short answer. *Nature* 24 May 2001;**411**(6836):428–9.

7   Selnes A, Bolle R, Holt J, Lund E. Cumulative incidence of asthma and allergy in north-Norwegian schoolchildren in 1985 and 1995. *Pediatr Allergy Immunol* 2002;**13**(1):58–63.

8   Custovic A, Murray CS, Gore RB, Woodcock A. Controlling indoor allergens. *Ann Allergy Asthma Immunol* 2002;**88**:432–41.

9   Custovic A, Simpson BM, Simpson A, Hallam C *et al.* Manchester Asthma and Allergy Study: low-allergen environment can be achieved and maintained during pregnancy and in early life. *J Allergy Clin Immunol* 2000;**105**;252–8.

10   Gotzsche PC, Johansen UK, Burr ML, Hammarquist C. House dust mite control measures for asthma. *Cochrane Database Systematic Rev* 2001; CD001187.

11   Custovic A, Simpson BM, Simpson A, Kissen P, Woodcock A. Effect of environmental manipulation in pregnancy and early life on respiratory symptoms and atopy during first year of life: a randomized trial. *Lancet* 2001;**358**:188–93.

12   Strachan DP. The role of environmental factors in asthma. *Br Med Bull* 2000;**56**:865–2.

13   Matricardi PM, Ronchetti R. Are infections protecting from atopy? *Curr Opin Allergy Clin Immunol* 2001;1:413–9.

14   Holt PG. Parasites, atopy, and the hygiene hypothesis: resolution of a paradox? *Lancet* 2000;**356**:1699–701.

15   Nahori MA, Lagranderie M, Lefort J, Thouron F *et al.* Effects of Mycobacterium bovis BCG on the development of allergic inflammation and bronchial hyperresponsiveness in hyper-IgE BP2 mice vaccinated as newborns. *Vaccine* 2001;**19**:1484–95.

16   Farooqi IS, Hopkin JM. Early childhood infection and atopic disorder. *Thorax.* 1998;**53**:927–32.

17 Pyama N, Sudo N, Sogawa H, Karbo C. Antibiotic use during infancy promotes Th-1/Th-2 balance towards Th-2 dominant immunity in mice. *J Allergy Clin Immunol* 2001;**107**:153–9.

18 Bjorksten B, Sepp E, Julge K, Voor T, Mikelsaar M. Allergy development and the intestinal microflora during the first year of life. *J Allergy Clin Immunol* 2001;**108**(4):516–20.

19 Malo JL, Chan-Yeung M. Occupational asthma. *J Allergy Clin Immunol* 2001;**108**:317–28.

20 Devereux G, Barker RN, Seaton A. Antenatal determinants of neonatal immune responses to allergens. *Clin Exp Allergy* 2002;**32**:43–50.

21 McConnell R, Berhane K, Gilliland F, London SJ *et al.* Asthma in exercising children exposed to ozone: a cohort study. *Lancet* 2002;**359**:386–91.

22 Hjern A, Hedberg A, Haglund B, Rosen M. Does tobacco smoke prevent atopic disorders? A study of two generations of Swedish residents. *Clin Exp Allergy* 2001;**31**(6):908–14.

23 Gdalevich M, Mimouni D, David M, Mimouni M. Breast-feeding and the onset of atopic dermatitis in childhood: a systematic review and meta-analysis of prospective studies. *J Am Acad Dermatol* 2001;**45**:520–7.

24 Varga EM, Durham SR. Allergen injection immunotherapy. *Clin Allergy Immunol* 2002;**16**:533–49.

Appendix 1
The burden of allergic disease in the UK

Introduction

Although allergy represents an important source of patient morbidity and healthcare utilisation, there is little reliable information on the overall disease burden posed by allergic conditions. However, a UK-based study was recently commissioned by the British Society for Allergy and Clinical Immunology (BSACI) to determine the prevalence of allergic conditions (excluding occupational allergy), to estimate the healthcare burden posed by these patients, and to assess recent disease trends in relation to the UK population.[1] Below is an overview of the data sources used, a description of the epidemiological and statistical methods employed, and a detailed presentation of the findings, together with a discussion of the possible implications of these findings for clinical care and health services planning. A short summary of the findings is provided in Chapter 2, Box 2.1, p 7.

Aims and objectives

The aim of the study was to quantify the healthcare burden posed by allergic diseases in the UK from 1991 to 2001, focusing on the following conditions: allergic rhinitis, anaphylaxis, asthma, conjunctivitis, eczema/dermatitis, food allergy and urticaria /angioedema. The objectives of the study were:

(1) to describe the prevalence, incidence and outcomes of these allergic disorders

(2) to describe the burden currently posed by allergic disorders to NHS primary and secondary care

(3) to estimate the health and societal costs of allergic disorders

(4) to comment on variations of allergic disease over time, by region and socio-economic status.

Methods

In order to maximise the generalisability of the results, analyses were confined to data from routine health information sources and large, high-quality, national and international surveys. These included:

▶ The Health Survey for England (HSE), Scottish Health Survey (SHS), International Study of Allergies and Asthma in Childhood (ISAAC) and the European Community Respiratory Health Survey (ECRHS) for estimates of symptomatic and clinician-diagnosed disease prevalence

▶ Morbidity Statistics from General Practice 1991/92 (MSGP4), Royal College of General

Practitioners Weekly Returns Service (RCGP WRS) and Prescribing Analysis and Cost (PACT) data for primary healthcare utilisation

▶ Hospital Episodes Statistics (HES) for data on hospital admissions.

Where data were not available from the above, reference is made to other high-quality studies.

Main findings

The main findings are summarised below in relation to the epidemiology of allergic conditions, healthcare utilisation, direct costs to the NHS, and disease trends. Data sources are indicated in parentheses.

Epidemiology

How common are allergic disorders in the UK?

Over one in three people in the UK have at some point in their lives been diagnosed with one or more allergic disorders (Fig. 1). Over 30% of the general population have at some point experienced symptoms of 'rhinoconjunctivitis', 'wheezing' and 'itchy skin', these being suggestive of diagnoses of allergic rhinitis, asthma and eczema (HSE).

When restricted to the previous 12 months, over 20% of children and adults will have experienced symptoms suggestive of allergic rhinitis, asthma and/or eczema (ECRHS, HSE, ISAAC). More than 3% of children are awake at night at least once a week from eczema and twice that number are woken at least once a week by wheeze (HSE).

Nearly 40% of children and 30% of adults have been diagnosed with one or more of the following: asthma, eczema and hay fever (HSE, ISAAC).

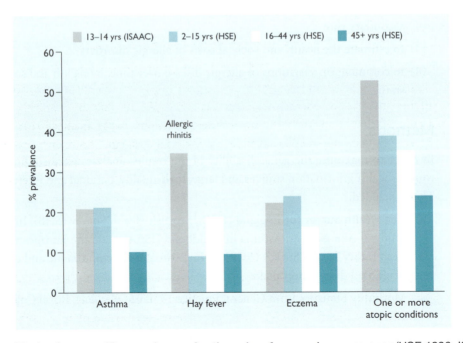

Fig 1   Age-specific prevalence of asthma, hay fever and eczema ever (HSE 1996, ISAAC UK).

Co-existing allergic disorders

Allergic problems frequently co-exist. Ten per cent of children (2–15 years) and young adults (16–44 years) have been diagnosed with more than one allergic disorder; 5% of older adults (over 45 years) have been diagnosed with more than one allergic condition (HSE). In series involving over 560 patients with nut allergy, 96% also had one or more of the following: allergic asthma (63%), allergic rhinitis (64%) and atopic eczema (61%).[2] Other food allergies also occurred.

How does UK prevalence of allergy compare with other countries?

The UK prevalence of symptoms suggestive of allergic rhinitis, asthma and eczema is amongst the highest in the world. Data on children from the 56 countries participating in the International Study of Asthma and Allergy in Children (ISAAC) showed that the UK ranked second with respect to eczema symptoms, third in relation to asthma symptoms and thirteenth in terms of rhinitis symptoms (ISAAC). Data on adults from the 17 countries participating in the European Community Respiratory Health Survey (ECRHS) survey showed that the UK ranked second in relation to rhinitis symptoms and third with respect to asthma symptoms (ECRHS).

What proportion of GP consultations are for allergic conditions?

Almost 6% of GP consultations are for allergic diseases. In 1991, GP consultation rates for allergic conditions were 21,200 per 100,000 patient years. Eczema, asthma and allergic rhinitis (in descending order of frequency) were the allergic conditions that most commonly necessitated GP consultation (MSGP4).

Overall, GP consultation rates for allergic conditions appear to have remained constant during the last decade. Mean weekly GP consultation rates in 2000 were 31.2, 29.3 and 21.2 per 100,000 for asthma, allergic rhinitis and eczema respectively (RCGP WRS).

What proportion of hospital admissions are for allergic conditions?

Approximately 0.6% of all NHS hospital admissions are for allergic diseases. However, this is almost certainly an underestimate, because allergy is frequently unrecognised. NHS hospital admission rates for allergic disorders were 92.5 per 100,000 in 2000/2001 (HES). Asthma accounted for the majority (87%) of these admissions. In the financial year 2000/2001 there were, however, over 9,000 admissions for other allergic problems (urticaria = 2,147; anaphylaxis = 1,964; atopic dermatitis = 1,528; food allergy = 1,388; allergic rhinitis = 1,156; angioedema = 819, and conjunctivitis = 90) (HES).

Costs to the NHS

How much does GP prescribed treatment for allergy cost the NHS?

Community prescribed treatments for allergic conditions cost the NHS £0.6 billion per annum (Fig. 2). Primary care prescribing costs for all conditions amount to £5.6 billion per annum. Treatments for allergic disorders including asthma currently account for 10% (£0.6 billion) of this budget (PACT). This figure is comparable to GP prescribing costs for gastrointestinal

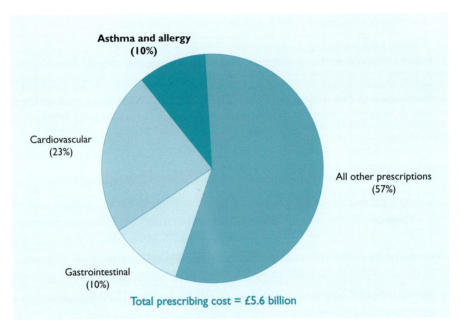

Total prescribing cost = £5.6 billion

Fig 2 Net ingredient costs of GP prescriptions for asthma and allergy compared to prescriptions for gastrointestinal and cardiovascular conditions (PACT).

disorders (10% of overall budget) and almost half that for cardiovascular conditions (23% of overall budget) (PACT).

How much do GP consultations and hospital admissions for allergy cost the NHS?

GP consultations and hospital admissions for allergic disease cost the NHS an estimated £283 million per annum. GP consultations for allergic problems cost an estimated £225 million per annum (MSGP4, RCGP WRS, Department of Health). Allergic problems are responsible for over 183,000 bed-days each year at an estimated cost of almost £58 million per annum (HES, Department of Health). Again, these figures will be underestimates.

Trends in disease frequency

What are the major trends in allergic disease frequency?

Allergic disease frequency appears to have increased substantially during recent decades (Fig. 3).

Asthma, rhinitis and eczema The prevalence of asthma, rhinitis and eczema have doubled or trebled in the last two decades in developed countries, including the UK. Between 1971 and 1991, GP consultation rates for asthma quadrupled, increasing from 960 per 100,000 patient years to 4,210 per 100,000 patient years (MSGP4). GP consultation rates for allergic rhinitis, more than doubled, increasing from 1,100 per 100,000 patient years to 2,830 per 100,000 patient years during the same time period (MSGP4). Patients consulting for eczema increased from 3,410 to 5,060/100,000 patient years between 1981 and 1991 (Source: MSGP4). During the last decade, primary care consultation rates for asthma, allergic rhinitis and eczema have begun to stabilise with little overall change between 1991 and 2000 (RCGP WRS).

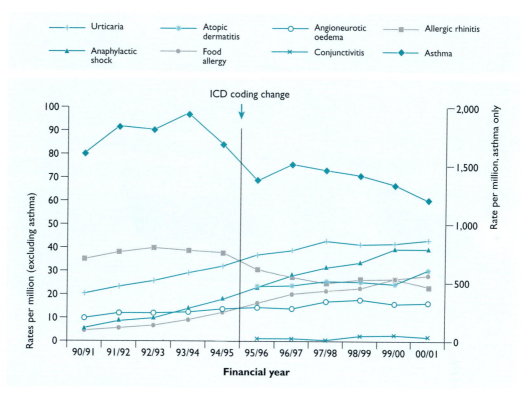

Fig 3   Trends in hospital admission rates for allergy (HES).

Food allergy   There is evidence of a substantial rise in peanut and nut allergy. Nut allergy was rare until the early 1990s; the first large series reported from a major allergy centre was in 1993–4; the incidence of peanut allergy in children in the UK was 0.5% in 1994 and had trebled to 1.6% four years later (ISAAC).[3,4,5]

Hospital admissions   Trends in hospital admissions for the time period 1990/91–2000/01 show year-on-year increases in admission rates for a range of systemic allergic conditions, including anaphylaxis, urticaria, angioedema and food allergy. Admissions for anaphylaxis, which account for a minority of cases (only the most severe), increased seven-fold over the last decade and doubled over four years.[6] Asthma admissions, however, declined during the latter half of the last decade (HES).

References

1   Gupta R, Sheikh A, Strachan DP, Anderson HR. The burden of allergic disease in the UK. Unpublished study (2002) commissioned by the British Society for Allergy and Clinical Immunology, London.

2   Ewan PW, Clark AT. Long-term prospective observational study of the outcome of a management plan in patients with peanut and nut allergy referred to a regional allergy centre. *Lancet* 2001;**357**:111–15.

3   Ewan PW. Clinical study of peanut and nut allergy in 62 consecutive patients: new features and associations. *BMJ* 1996;**312**:1074–8.

4   Tariq SM, Stevens M, Matthews W, Ridout S *et al.* Cohort strudy of peanut and tree nut sensitisation by age of 4 years. *BMJ* 1996;**313**:514–7.

5   Grundy J, Matthews S, Bateman B, Dean T, Arshad SH. Rising prevalence of allergy to peanut in children: data from 2 sequential cohorts. *J Allergy Clin Immunol* 2002;**110**:784–9.

6   Sheikh A, Alves B Hospital admissions for acute anaphylaxis: time trend study. *BMJ* 2000;**320**:1441.

Appendix 2
Useful addresses

The British Society for Allergy and Clinical Immunology (BSACI) is the professional body representing allergists. It publishes a handbook of *National Health Service Allergy Clinics*, a comprehensive and regularly updated list, describing the nature of allergy services provided.
PO Box 35649, London SE9 1WA.
Tel: 020 8859 6118 Website: www.bsaci.org

UK allergy charities

The charities listed below are independent bodies and their inclusion in this document does not imply endorsement by the Royal College of Physicians.

Allergy UK is a patient support organisation with a broad sphere of interest, encompassing various types of allergy and intolerance.
Deepdene House, 30 Bellegrove Road, Welling, Kent DA16 3PY.
Helpline: 020 8303 8583. Website: www.allergyfoundation.com

The Anaphylaxis Campaign is a patient support organisation focusing on potentially life-threatening allergic reactions.
PO Box 275, Farnborough, Hampshire GU14 6SX.
Helpline: 01252 542029. Website: www.anaphylaxis.org.uk

The Latex Allergy Support Group provides support for people affected by latex allergy and their families.
PO Box 27, Filey YO14 9YH.
Helpline (7pm–10pm): 07071 225838. Website: www.lasg.co.uk

The MedicAlert Foundation is a non-profit-making registered charity providing a life-saving identification system for individuals with hidden medical conditions and allergies.
1 Bridge Wharf, 156 Caledonian Road, London N1 9UU.
Tel: 020 7833 3034. Website: www.medicalert.org.uk

The National Asthma Campaign provides information on asthma management for asthma sufferers.
Providence House, Providence Place, London N1 0NT.
Helpline: 0845 7 01 02 03. Website: www.asthma.org.uk

The National Eczema Society provides education and training for eczema sufferers.
Hill House, Highgate Hill, London N19 5NA.
Helpline: 0870 241 3604. Website: www.eczema.org